THE
BOY WHO
GAVE HIS
HEART
AWAY

THE
BOY WHO
GAVE HIS
HEART
AWAY

*A Death that Brought
the Gift of Life*

COLE MORETON

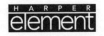

HarperElement
An imprint of HarperCollins*Publishers*

ISBN 978-0-00-822572-8

Printed and bound in Great Britain by
Clays Ltd, St Ives plc

MIX
Paper from
responsible sources
FSC C007454

FSC™ is a non-profit international organisation established to promote
the responsible management of the world's forests. Products carrying the
FSC label are independently certified to assure consumers that they come
from forests that are managed to meet the social, economic and
ecological needs of present and future generations,
and other controlled sources.

Find out more about HarperCollins and the environment at
www.harpercollins.co.uk/green

INTRODUCTION

This is the true story of two boys who never met, but who are bound together in the most astonishing way. Marc was fit and fast, a star player in his local football team. Strong and brave but shy and gentle, he had a sharp face, sandy hair and striking green eyes. Martin was big, bright and breezy, a loving lad who was always up for a laugh, with a mop of brown hair and a friendly face that made everyone smile. Their names were alike and they were more or less the same age, either side of a sixteenth birthday, but they lived hundreds of miles apart in Scotland and England and never even knew each other existed. Then, one summer, they both fell down. Just like that, without warning, they were taken seriously ill at the same time. That's where we begin. One of these boys will die. And without ever knowing it, he will save the other's life.

This is also the story of their mums, Linda and Sue, who will go through grief and worry enough to break most of us. I have got to know the families, the medics and one of the boys well over several years and this book is based on their own accounts of what happened, which are terribly sad but also inspirational and full of wonders. Towards the end of the telling, the mother of the boy who was lost will meet the boy who was saved, now grown into a man. She will reach out and put her hand flat against his chest, to feel the heart of her own poor son still beating away inside him. Life will have sprung from death, miraculously. But before that extraordinary moment can happen, there must be a tragedy. Marc or Martin. One of these boys is about to give his heart away ...

We are not meant to touch hearts. Hearts are away, hidden, at the centre where they can't be got at. Protected. Vital. The seat of the soul. If a heart is touched, it can only be a miracle.

Louisa Young, The Book of the Heart *2002*

ONE

MARC

Marc was in agony, writhing around on the back seat of the car and calling for his mum. She was driving as fast as she could, up to the hospital and over the red warning lines, straight into the ambulance bay, blocking the way for everyone else. Linda didn't care. She thought her son was dying. She was right. She leaned on the horn again and again and the loud, flat sound echoed under the canopy, an alarm and a plea for help. 'Come out! Come on! Where are you?'

Marc couldn't walk and there was no way she could carry a hefty, dazed teenager out of the car and all the way through the doors to Accident & Emergency, but surely somebody in there would hear the noise and wonder what was going on? A hospital porter came striding over with an angry face but

Linda shouted at him: 'I'm not moving. Not until my son gets seen!'

The porter was confused, he knew her as a friend and a nurse who worked the night shift. Then he looked into the back of the car and saw Marc in a terrible state.

'Holy crap, Linda – is that your boy?'

Yanking open the car door, he swore loudly and waved at a colleague for a trolley. Marc didn't answer his questions and Linda couldn't get the words out right. 'Just help him, please.'

The porter took hold of Marc under both arms to lift him out and tried to be reassuring. 'We'll take him, hen. You get this thing moved, yeah?'

Linda turned the key, put her foot down and the car lurched forward out of the bay. She left it half up on a pavement and ran back through the double doors into the gloomy reception area where the faces of the sick and injured looked up at her. Where the hell was Marc?

'This way,' shouted a voice she knew and Linda saw the fuss around her son first. A couple of nurses in blue, busy with machines and a tangle of wires and tubing. More coming over. A young doctor in a white coat saying something about the lad being only fifteen. Marc was on the trolley in the middle of the growing crowd, already with a clear plastic breathing mask over his face and then Linda knew – she just knew, in her shock and horror – that this was as serious as it could be.

'My poor wee man is dying away …'

'When the sun shone his hair went blonder. He had lovely green eyes, just like his father,' says Linda now, sitting cross-legged on a sofa and remembering Marc as a child. Her hands turn over and over on her lap, a little sign of anguish. 'Marc was a quiet boy. A shy boy. The best boy ever.' The mothers and fathers of children who have been in danger or lost often say things like that, but they are not deluding themselves. It's self-defence. If mums didn't forget the pain of giving birth, no more babies would be born. In the same way, we try to forget how scary it is to be a parent. We wrap the good times around us instead, for protection. 'He had the best nature of all my children,' says Linda in her urgent, breathy voice with a strong Scottish accent. 'Any one of the others will tell you that.'

She had only just turned forty when Marc fell ill in the summer of 2003, but Linda already had four sons and a daughter aged between thirteen and nineteen. The kids had been raised in the beautiful countryside west of Glasgow but they now lived with her or close to each other in houses and flats around Johnstone, a town struggling for an identity. Linda loved being a mum, and thank God for that she says with a laugh. 'I'd been pregnant for the whole of the Eighties!'

The family name is McCay, to rhyme with hay. She was no longer married to Norrie, the father of her children – a sharp, funny guy who worked as a roofer – but Linda still used his name and he was still in all their lives. 'Together or apart, divorced or not, we were good parents.'

Linda worked four nights a week as a nursing assistant at the Royal Alexandra Hospital in Paisley, a few miles from Johnstone. She relied on her mother and daughter for help with the young ones. 'We all hung out together, we were still a close family.' The boys supported Rangers, the proud old Glasgow club. Ryan, the second eldest lad, was a professional footballer heading for the Scottish Premier League and Marc wanted to get there too, so he played the game any time he could: at school, on the field, at midweek training, in the league on Saturday when the scouts from the big clubs were watching, at the park with his mates on Sunday, anywhere. Kicking and running, shooting and scoring. Banging them in. He was strong and fast up front – the top scorer in his team – a fit lad with a good pair of shoulders and a sharp face under his fringe of sandy hair. He could have made it, says Linda. 'A lot of people said Marc was a better footballer than his brother. He was a happy lad, chasing his dream. Then a virus came and attacked him, out of the blue.'

Marc was fine when he went away with his big brother Darren that summer, to an all-inclusive resort in Ibiza. Boys will be boys and Linda didn't dare ask too many questions, but their texts got a bit worrying. 'The last couple of days he was a bit breathless and said he was having terrible pains in his tummy. I thought maybe he'd caught a bug. I remember standing at Glasgow Airport and seeing him come through to Arrivals. He looked yellow, there was something really not right with him.'

The ache in his bones felt like the flu and the stomach pains drove him to his bed. Linda worried that her son's liver was failing – she had seen the signs at work – but Marc insisted he had barely touched a drop of alcohol on holiday. His brother backed him up and she believed them both. He was that keen on being fit for the football. 'I never thought it was really the drink, not for a moment. Alarm bells were ringing in my head. I was thinking, "What's going on here?"'

Linda left Marc lying on the sofa at home listless the next day, watching television, not eating and complaining of the pain, which wasn't like him at all. Then she heard groaning and found him tossing about in a fever, unable to take in what she was saying to him. 'He was even more yellow, a horrible colour. And he was confused. It was as though the light was on and nobody was in, he was so disorientated.'

The locum they saw at the family clinic that afternoon decided Marc had overdone it on holiday, drunk too much or taken whatever lads took at his age. Marc swore otherwise but the doctor didn't believe him. 'Go home and rest. Take painkillers. Eat healthy and drink plenty of fluids and you'll be fine.' But Marc wasn't fine. As soon as they got outside the clinic he wandered off up the street, staggering about like a drunk.

'Come here, son …'

'What?'

He sounded confused. Then he bent over double, crying and shouting, growling with the pain. Scared, Linda thought fast. She didn't want to go back into the clinic and face that doctor again. An ambulance could take ages. The hospital was only a couple of miles outside Johnstone, so she got Marc to the car somehow, holding him up all the way.

'I felt very frustrated, very angry.'

He let her lay him down on the back seat. 'He was just exhausted and putting his life into my hands: "Mum is telling me to lie down, so I will lie down."'

Traffic lights and roundabouts slowed them down on the way to the Royal Alexandra Hospital, on a hill just outside of town. Linda was torn between wanting to put her foot down and go fast between the lights – to hell with the speed limit – and not wanting to throw her fragile boy about too much.

'Sorry, son. Sorry …'

The car park was full and it was too far from the entrance in any case, but the ambulance bay at A&E was empty. Cars were banned but she went for it anyway. 'I am a very pushy person and for once in my life that was an advantage. I don't know if it was mother's instinct or the experience I had of seeing people in that hospital who were very ill, but I knew my son was in deep, deep trouble.'

Linda had seen parents in the ward demented with fear, their faces all wet with tears, and now it was her turn. She knew the doctors and nurses here – their first names, their little habits and irritations, how they behaved under pressure – so she saw how baffled they were by his test results.

'What is happening to my son?'

'Linda, I've got to be honest,' said a doctor. 'We just don't know.'

Marc's liver was failing, they told her, but his other organs were suffering too. His life was in danger, but they could not be sure of the cause. He would have to go to the Royal Infirmary of Edinburgh straight away, for more expert help. Linda went all the way to the door of the ambulance with her son, who was unconscious on the trolley as the medics lifted him in. There was not enough room for her with all the equipment Marc needed, they were very sorry. She felt a terrible aching and a longing as she watched the white and yellow ambulance leave the hospital that Wednesday evening, 20 August 2003, with the blue light flashing and the siren telling everyone to get out of the way.

Her boy was being taken away, beyond her outstretched arms. How could she hold him close and safe now?

TWO

MARTIN

Three hundred miles to the south, another teenage boy was playing football in the park. A friendly lad with a wide, gap-toothed smile and a mop of brown hair, Martin Burton was just having a kick-about with his mates in the warmth of a late summer evening in Grantham, Lincolnshire. He wore a West Ham United shirt, partly to wind up his big brother who supported Forest, but Martin was too much of a gentle soul to be properly sporty. He had a fuzz of hair on his top lip and was rapidly growing out of his puppy fat into the hefty build of a centre-back, having just turned sixteen. Emotionally, he was still young for his age though. Martin was a bit of a softie on the quiet, in a nice way. His bed was covered in soft toys he called 'cuddlies', brought home by his father Nigel from many trips away with the Royal Air Force.

'From the day he was born he was always noisy, he was always in your face,' says his mother Sue, a quiet and reserved English costs lawyer who was in her early forties. 'He was a "Boy" with a capital B; but he was also a very caring and loving child and a really good friend. Martin was very popular and always helping people. His headmaster said he had a lot to say but he was never in any real trouble, and if the teacher needed any help then his hand was the first to go up.' Martin told great stories, but something misfired when he tried to write things down. 'They tested him for dyslexia, because he wasn't just lazy. He did have a struggle with schooling, but they never could find any reason for that.'

His ambition was to be a nurse and everyone agreed he would be great but his GCSE results a week or so earlier had not been good enough. 'Martin wasn't an academic, he was just a boy who loved life. He was too busy having fun to concentrate on what he should have been doing, I'm afraid. His attitude to school was, "I've turned up every day for 12 years, what more do they want?"' So Martin was going to engineering college instead. 'He was better with his hands. I'm very good with my hands,' says Nigel Burton, who was a senior aircraft technician in the RAF.

For now, though, Martin could enjoy the sweltering days of late August with his friends. He was fit and happy, says his mum. 'There was absolutely no sign whatsoever that anything was about to go wrong.'

THREE

MARC

The long, bright corridors of the newly rebuilt Royal Infirmary of Edinburgh could have been the set of an American medical drama. Linda McCay wandered them in the early hours of the morning, not really knowing or caring where she was going, clutching a Bible tight to her chest and praying out loud for her boy.

'Please don't take my son. I'll do anything you want. I'm sorry for everything bad I've done in the past. I will be a better person. I'll not smoke …'

Her blonde hair was tangled like a bird's nest after being twisted and pulled over the six days and nights she had kept up a vigil for Marc in that large, intimidating new hospital on the edge of the city. Sometimes she cried and walked until morning. Sometimes she sat in the chapel. Sometimes she slumped in a chair in a corner somewhere, oblivious to a passing trolley with its urgent crew of attendants or a weary nurse coming off shift who had taken too much crap that night to intrude – and sometimes Linda just prayed and had no idea what else she was doing. 'Please. Anything. I promise, I promise …'

In front of her, a man thumped the vending machine with the flat of his hand, cursing. Linda recognised him as one of the doctors in the team trying to keep her son alive, a crumpled figure in need of an iron for his shirt but with an air of authority. There were bags under the bags under his eyes, but she knew Marc's life depended on him and his colleagues. The doctor gave up on the machine for a moment and offered Linda a weak, weary, sympathetic smile.

'Your son has been unlucky. Very unlucky indeed.'

A virus had probably attacked Marc while he was on holiday in Ibiza. Maybe a snotty kid had wiped his runny nose with the back of a hand, before leaving an invisible smear on a table top or a drinking glass. The little boy would never have known he was a carrier. A fever was easy to miss in a hot place, if you were in and out of the pool all day. Anyone could have come along and picked up the virus in that smear but it was Marc who did so, perhaps as he took a drink or lay down a poker card on the table. Maybe he put his fingers to his mouth just then, absent-mindedly. Maybe he stopped a sneeze. Maybe his eye was irritated by a trace of sun cream, so he rubbed it. Either way, the bug entered his body. That was when his luck turned really bad.

Most people catch a cold or a sore throat from the same virus but after a few days the body fights it off and the bad feeling passes. This time the cells of the virus travelled through the bloodstream all the way to the meaty muscle of Marc's heart. This is the myocardium and a bad attack by a virus leaves it thin and inflamed, a rare condition known as acute viral myocarditis. We don't pay that meaty muscle much attention, but it is the practical reason we go on living, the engine room of our ship, the physical source of the power that keeps our lights on. Ba-boom, ba-boom, ba-boom. That's the rhythm of life, the sound of the engine working, pumping blood into the lungs to pick up the oxygen we need to survive, then pumping it on again to feed the rest of the body.

When the engine fails, we know it. The lights go out.

Marc's heart was ill and swollen and could beat only weakly so the blood was not getting around his body properly. His organs were being starved of the oxygen they needed and they were failing – his liver was drying up, his lungs filling with blood. Marc was fading fast.

His family took turns to stand by his bedside, watching over him. Leasa, his sister, who was just nineteen and studying to be a nurse, had read that if you cry in front of people who are unconscious they might hear you and get scared, but if you tell them stories or sing it might stimulate their brain. So she sang to him. The song that came to mind was called Pretty Green Eyes by Ultrabeat and it usually had a massive club sound; but as she sat there by his bedside in the quiet murmur of the hospital, singing into his ear, her pure, clear voice made it sound like a song as old as the hills.

Pretty green eyes,
So full of wonder and despair,
It's all right to cry, for I'll be there to wipe your
*   tears …*
You'll never have to be alone.

Blood is pumped away from the heart to the rest of the body through the arteries and one of them runs deep through the groin and the leg. For the doctors, it offers a way into places that are otherwise untouchable without surgery. They injected Marc with a long needle and pushed an impossibly thin, flexible pipe through the needle, into the artery and all the way up his body against the flow of blood, into his chest. Gas was used to inflate and deflate a six-inch-long balloon on the end of the pipe so that it rose and fell inside the aorta – the main artery of the body – with a natural rhythm to match that of the heart, allowing the inflamed and weary muscle to rest and recover its strength. Amazing … but it wasn't enough.

Marc's heart was too damaged and weak for the balloon to help much, so they tried a more advanced piece of kit that was new to the Royal Infirmary: a device that sucked blood out of the body, gave it oxygen and pumped it back in – a bedside mechanical stand-in for the heart and lungs. This was cutting-edge technology that made the television news that evening: 'For the first time ever in Scotland, a mechanical assist has been used to keep a patient's heart going.' And it was a fantastic success at first. The monitors that had been so quiet as Marc lay there, barely functioning, now bleeped and flashed as his body found new strength.

Norrie, Marc's father, who was a roofer in his forties at the time, remembers what he said when he saw the screens behind Marc come to life: 'Wow, this is us sorted. It's like the Blackpool Illuminations in here!'

Linda was in the room with him and she was just as thrilled. She grabbed hold of her ex-husband and laughed, but the joy didn't last. The movement on the monitors slowed again and then stopped, and within half an hour they were as quiet as before. Marc was sinking again. And the high was followed by a new low. Linda saw something else now, something that horrified her. She noticed that the colour had begun to drain from Marc's legs, leaving them grey with white and red blotches. The death tartan. She recognised that from seeing patients die on her ward.

'That's it, he's going now,' she thought, getting angry. 'This is not the way the world is meant to work. They are not supposed to go before us!'

So says every parent who has had to watch a child die. Stunned and confused, she and Norrie went back to the family room, where their sons and daughter and Linda's mother did not know what to say. Then the doctor entered the room too and the sky fell in.

'Marc is dying right now, as we speak, and there is nothing else we can do.'

Linda heard a fierce sound like a riot in the street outside, but it was right beside her: Betty, her 'wee, sensible mother', going frantic. Linda heard her cries through the double glazing of panic and fear. Norrie was angry too, but their daughter Leasa tried to hold it all together for all of them. The eldest and quietest child was also the strongest, and now as the doctor talked again about a virus and tried to explain myocarditis she interrupted him and the words came spilling out of her. 'What does that mean? He's fit, he's healthy, he doesn't drink and he doesn't smoke. We've got no history of heart problems in the family. What are you talking about?'

She thought of her brother, wrapped in silver foil to keep the heat in as warm air was fanned over his body, and Leasa felt as if the doctors had already made their decision and all this medical jargon was a way to justify letting him go. 'It was like they were giving him his last rites.'

Linda lost control then and in her wild panic she fixed on a consultant cardiologist who had come to help explain, a small man she thought looked Italian. Grabbing his lapels, she yelled into his face. 'You've got to do something. He's only fifteen!' The doctor was sorry, he said. He told them that he would do anything he could to save Marc, she had to believe that, but that they had run out of options.

'There is nothing more we can do.'

What do you say when your friend is dying? How do you go up to a mate in a coma, all wrapped up in blankets, unconscious with a tube down his throat and all those wires connecting his body to machines, in front of his parents and his granny and his sister, and say, 'Yeah, so … Right. Goodbye then, pal.' The two lads who came to visit Marc were brave and resourceful but they couldn't help the tears. Linda held them both, one on either side of her, pushing their heads hard against her shoulders as if trying to squeeze the pain away, for all three of them. It didn't work.

Norrie was in the corner of the room, answering strange questions from the dishevelled but commanding doctor: 'What height is Marc? What weight do you think he is?'

Linda overheard and turned on the medic, furiously. 'What are you asking that for? You wanna be measuring him for the morgue, is that it?'

'No, Linda, hang on,' said Norrie, grabbing a hand to get her to listen. 'There's something going on, they've got an idea, I'm sure of it.'

She refused to believe it until the doctor offered just a chance, the slimmest chance, of help. 'There is a machine in Newcastle, it could take over the work of Marc's heart and keep him going until another heart becomes available.'

'What do you mean?'

'From a donor.'

A dead boy's heart. Or a girl's. A dead girl's heart in Marc – that struck Linda as even stranger for a moment. But then again, why not? 'Could it be anyone?'

'As long as the size and blood type are right. You won't remember this I'm sure, of course – there's a lot going on for you – but this machine is called an ECMO, or extracorporeal membrane oxygenation machine ...'

Weirdly, those words stayed in Linda's brain forever, as did the next thing she heard the doctor say. '... Make no mistake, Marc is dying right now. There is only a one per cent chance he can survive the journey. He might not even make it off the hospital bed and down that corridor, let alone all the way to Newcastle ...'

'What did you say, about Marc's chances?'

'One per cent. I'm sorry, Norrie, I can't put it higher than that.'

Norrie seized the tiny chance anyway. 'What are we waiting for? Let's go now!'

But Linda hesitated – she looked down at her son – she understood what was likely to happen. 'If my son dies in that ambulance he is going to die on his own, isn't he? He needs us with him. Please let me and his dad go with him.'

The doctor was touched, Linda could see that, but she remembers being told it was not possible. They were going to use a specialist intensive care ambulance to take Marc to Edinburgh Airport, where he would be put on an adapted plane and flown down to Newcastle. There was already barely enough room in the ambulance for the medical staff and all the equipment they needed to fight for Marc's life. A police escort would take spare oxygen bottles for the ventilator, but one person might be able to squeeze in there and then sit in the back of the plane if it was big enough. That was the best they could do. Another ambulance and patrol car would be waiting when they landed. Norrie said he would go with the cops, if they let him. Leasa, the level-headed daughter, took control of her mum. 'You're better off coming in the car with me. We'll go down together.'

Linda was terrified. She was panicking and pleading in her head, praying, 'God, can I make a deal, make a pact?' Then she got an idea so crazy that she thought it just might work. She grabbed the doctor's arm tight and yanked him, demanding his full attention. 'Listen, I'm forty, I've had my life, can you not give Marc my heart, here and now?'

She meant it, too. They could have put Linda under with anaesthetic right there and then and taken a knife to her chest, pulled out her heart to give to Marc and left her dead and she would have let it happen, without hesitation.

'I'm serious, I'm telling you, why not?

'Please, doctor, please. Please give my heart to my son.'

They couldn't. Of course not. No doctor would kill a healthy mother to save an ailing, almost-adult son, no matter how much she pleaded. The others all knew that.

'Come on, Mum. Come on,' said Leasa, pulling her close. So once again Linda had to let her boy go, despite every instinct telling her that this journey would be his last, feeling that prayers were all she had left.

'Please, God. Don't let him die on the way.'

FOUR

MARTIN

Hot and sweaty from playing football and thirsty for milk from the fridge, Martin Burton got back to his house in Grantham on that Tuesday evening to find there was nobody else home. His big brother was at his girlfriend's house for tea and would spend the night there. He already knew his mother Sue was at the swimming pool with her friend. Martin had eaten his dinner before going off to the park but now he wanted a big bowl of Coco Pops. If he ate a bit too much sometimes, well then he burned it off. A restless lad, he was always on the go and up for a laugh. The telephone rang and it was his father calling from America, where he was on a desert exercise with the RAF. It was a happy, chatty call of the kind they always had when Dad was away.

'Am I going to get a cuddly?'

'Sorry son. You've got plenty. This isn't a cuddly place – they don't have a lot of cuddlies in Las Vegas.'

It was no big deal, he always asked that. They laughed about it then said goodnight.

'Love you, son.'

'Love you, Dad.'

However many miles were between them, they were still close. Nigel was a military man but his sons meant the world to him.

When the call was over, Martin probably turned up the television louder than Mum usually allowed, because he didn't like to be on his own. *Big Brother* was his favourite, all those people going mad in a house like a prison, only it looked fun with the stuff they had to do, dressing up and playing silly games. A big lad in a kilt called Cameron had just won it a month before and he was nice. Martin bounded up to his mum for a hug when she came in from swimming, her hair still wet. They sat together for a while watching the box, his legs over hers. This was a bit uncomfortable because Martin was a growing boy of sixteen and she was petite – 'but you've got to enjoy having them close while you can, haven't you?' That was what she always said. Her other son had grown up so fast and, proud as she was of the man he was becoming, she missed him as a boy. Nothing was wrong with Martin that night. Nothing at all. She left him watching the telly and went to bed. 'Be quiet when you come up, will you? I've got work in the morning.'

Sue was a small, neat woman with a short dark hair, serious glasses and an efficient manner. She liked an orderly home, which was a challenge with teenagers. Still, they knew very well that they were loved by their mum. She had flashes of temper about things like leaving dirty washing all over the floor but Mum also knew how to have fun. They lived in a detached house with a garage and a drive on the edge of Grantham, a quiet market town in the flatlands of Lincolnshire, best known as the birthplace of the former Prime Minister Margaret Thatcher, not that there was much to show for it. Grantham didn't like to make a fuss, and the Burtons were a bit like that too.

They had moved to the town when Nigel was stationed at a local airbase. It seemed sensible to buy a house and make a family home somewhere, rather than travel all over the world after him. Nigel had been to war once in the Balkans and twice in the Gulf since then, but the boys were safe and settled in Grantham. Now their youngest was just on the verge of becoming a man, says Sue. 'Martin was just getting to the age when boys gain maturity and he had started to be a bit more sensible. Girls had come on the scene. There was a big gang of boys and girls who used to hang around together. His body and his personality were changing. When he went to bed he was a normal, happy teenager.'

Sue woke at two in the morning because of the noise – there was a lot of banging and bumping coming from Martin's room across the landing. This wasn't fair, she had to get up early for work. 'Martin? What on earth are you doing?'

She sat up in bed just as her son appeared in the doorway, a silhouette in the dark. He looked strange in the half light, but she couldn't say why. Martin looked into the room at his mum but somehow looked right through her, as if he couldn't see or recognise her face. 'Martin?' His answer was just a mumble. Was this one of his jokes? Had he fallen out of bed and banged his head?

'What's the matter, love? Stop pratting about!'

He mumbled again and took a couple of steps forward but his knees buckled and he collapsed, face down, on her bed. Frightened now, she shook him but he slid off and rolled onto the floor.

'Get up! Come on!'

But Martin was slumped against the side of the bed in his pyjamas, the shirt riding up. His mother touched his face and it was warm but not fevered. She stroked his hair once, maybe twice, trying to be calm but feeling the fear rising as she wondered what on earth to do. The only phone was across the landing in the spare room so she ran in there to phone for an ambulance, calling back, 'Hang on, love. Hang on.'

'Is he breathing?' the emergency operator wanted to know, so Sue rushed back to check, rolling Martin into the recovery position as best she could. He was a big lad. Breathing, yes. With a guttural noise like a deep snore that scared her. 'That's when I realised it was serious. He wasn't getting up. But it still never entered my mind that this could be life-threatening.'

The operator was clear and precise. 'Okay, can you open the bedroom curtains please and put the light on so the ambulance driver can see which house in the street is yours? Then I need you to go downstairs and unlock the front door, is that okay?'

The ambulance arrived within minutes.

'I saw the flashing lights outside from the room upstairs. I called from the top of the stairs and they came up. They shone a light into his eyes, asked me what had happened and got him straight on to a stretcher.'

Sue pulled on a T-shirt and some jeans and found her purse and keys. 'They wouldn't let me in the ambulance until they were ready, but they did say, "Have you locked the door? Have you got your phone? You're going to need to make some calls." All the practical things they are trained to say, I guess. They wanted to make sure I was leaving the place secure. I just wanted to go.'

She rode in the ambulance with her son, holding on hard as it swayed around corners. 'This was two in the morning now and the Grantham hospital was only two miles from our house, so it took minutes, literally. Martin looked fast asleep. They got him out of the ambulance and into the hospital, then they were like, "The waiting room is over there ..." They whizzed him off through some doors, which promptly slammed behind him, shutting me out. I was stuck in the waiting room, the only person there. There was not even anybody behind the desk because it was the middle of the night and the main doors were locked.'

There were no other patients waiting to be seen, the little hospital was empty. The hard plastic seat pinched the back of her legs. She shivered. This was the quiet time between the last of the drunks and the first of the morning casualties. The calm before the dawn. The moments piled up, crowding her in. Sue was getting cold and scared but she was made of strong stuff. This will all work out, she told herself. No need to panic. 'Somebody came and took notes: name and address, date of birth, allergies and that sort of thing. Then some young doctor came and asked me, was there a chance Martin had taken any drugs? I was pretty sure the answer was no.'

The doctor was insistent: 'What about his brother, would he know? Could we perhaps ring him, just to make sure?'

'No, we cannot,' said Sue, rattled. Christopher had just turned twenty, he was sleeping over at his girl-friend Ashley's house, his mother did not think it was appropriate to disturb him. 'Unless you have got good reason to believe it's drugs, I'm not waking Christopher to ask him.'

So then she was left alone again, on her own in the empty waiting room. Her mouth was dry, her eyes felt raw. A nurse came after a while and asked if she wanted to ring someone and ask them to come over to the hospital, but Sue said no. 'I'm a Forces wife. I'm a big girl, I've spent a lot of my married life on my own, I'm used to handling things. I am not waking anyone at this hour just because my son has bumped his head.'

The nurse returned at four in the morning and insisted it would actually be best to call someone, to have them there for support. 'Martin really is very poorly.'

That was when the penny dropped, remembers Sue. 'She was drip-feeding me. This was the first time anyone had said that it was really serious.' But the nurse was not going to tell her just how serious it was until there was someone to hold her hand. Or to catch her fall.

The phone rang and rang until the answerphone clicked on. 'Please leave a message after the tone.' Sue pressed redial and listened again to the purr of the call, steady and insistent, alerting the landline in the house of her parents, Len and Joan, in Lincoln, twenty-five miles to the north. If they didn't pick up, what was she going to do? Who else could she call? Could she get the police to go round there and rouse them?

'Hello?'

Her father sounded startled.

'Dad, it's me, Sue. Listen, I need you –'

'Who is this?'

He was confused by sleep. She got frustrated and shouted.

'It's Susan. Your daughter. I'm in hospital –'

'What's wrong? Are you hurt? Where are you?'

'It's Martin. He's had a fall. I need you to come, Dad. I'm on my own …'

The confusion fell away as Len recognised what she was saying and the fear in her voice woke him up, fully. 'We'll be there as soon as we can.' He shook Joan, they dressed quickly and set off in the chill of the early morning. Both were seventy-three years old.

Len was concentrating on the road but Joan was worried, really worried. 'What did she say exactly? Come on, she must have said more than that? What do you think is wrong? Did she really give you no idea?' The sky began to glow beyond the street lights during the forty-minute drive. The roads were empty. The world seemed calm, too calm.

They were both scared stiff but Len was trying not to think too much about what was happening as they arrived at the hospital, a huddle of low prefab buildings that looked more like an old army base. They had to press a buzzer to be let into the hospital, which was otherwise deserted.

Sue was in a back room, distraught. 'They think he's got a bleed on his brain. They're taking him to Nottingham to see a specialist, right away.'

The nurse beside her spoke softly. 'Would you like to see him before he goes?'

Sue felt giddy, fluttery. 'Yes, please.'

'He's on a machine …'

Somewhere in among the nurses and the monitors and drips and tubes in a room full of people and things was Martin. Her normal instinct would have been to push everyone aside, but Sue was rattled by what was happening and uncertain of herself in that moment: the doctors must know best. So she held back, thinking, 'I have to let them do whatever they need to do.'

But then the nurses parted and she saw Martin, under a clear plastic mask. His eyes were closed. His hair was all messed up. He was unusually still, she sensed that in an instant. She hoped he couldn't hear all this commotion: the beeping of the monitors, the tense conversations between staff, the rattling of her own heart. He would be afraid, poor love. She moved in close, trying to reassure him. 'You've had a fall. That's all, silly pudding. You've bumped your head. You'll be fine.'

There was no way of knowing if he could hear her voice, but she had to say something, even if she was struggling to believe it. Half-blind from the tears, Sue bent to give her son a brief, soft kiss on the forehead before he was taken to the ambulance. 'It's all right, love. It's all right. Mum's here. Everything will be okay.'

FIVE

MARC

Marc was not going to make it down the corridor. He could not survive being moved out of the ward in a swarm of medics, trailing drips, monitors and machines. If he did then he would die in the lift on the way down to the specialist ambulance or somewhere out on the City of Edinburgh bypass in the night. There was no way he would get to the airport alive, his mum and dad were convinced of that, although neither of them dared say so. They were both hoping and praying to be wrong. Linda was weeping and keening as the bed was loaded into a big, boxy white ambulance. Marc lay at the centre of an octopus of tubes and wires. The ventilator was helping his lungs, the mechanical assist relieving his heart. All of this was tricky to get into the vehicle and it was going to be even harder to move out and into the aircraft without a slip that could mean a broken connection and a nasty death. They had to get there first, though. One of the medics, a stubbled Scot who might have had a son of his own about the same age, flashed Norrie McCay a sympathetic look. Norrie hoped he would talk to Marc on the way, even though the boy was unconscious. He didn't want his son to feel alone.

'Come on, son, let's do this,' Norrie said to himself as he got into the back of the police escort car, as if he was talking to Marc. But when they pulled up on the apron at Edinburgh Airport, he could see a problem. A really serious one.

'Is that the plane for our Marc?'

'Aye,' said his driver. 'Think so.'

Norrie had imagined a transporter plane that would open up at the back and allow the ambulance to drive right in – but this was just a small light aircraft, nowhere near big enough for the equipment, Marc and the medics. It was horrifying.

'I'd no get in that door myself. What the hell's going on? My Marc's dying here!'

'Calm down. We'll get this sorted.'

The police officers looked uncertain as they went into a huddle with the ambulance crew on the tarmac. Norrie listened with the window of the police car wound down then called his oldest child, Leasa, on his mobile. 'They're saying the plane's too small, hen.'

He was beginning to panic now. The one per cent chance of survival he had grabbed so thankfully and desperately was vanishing. 'They've got tae take us by road. No, I don't understand it either.'

Norrie remembers being told there was only enough battery power in the ambulance to keep the life-saving machines in the back going without a recharge for another two hours. The Freeman Hospital in Newcastle was at least two and a half hours away by the usual route, down the A1 through Berwick, Seahouses and Alnwick and into the city from the north. There was not enough time, even at night. This was hopeless, but the driver had a plan. They could go a more direct way, cross-country down the A68, shaving off miles. This might be a rollercoaster ride over the border hills, but if the police car went ahead to clear the way they hoped to drive smoothly enough to keep from hurting Marc. They might just make it before the power in the medical systems began to run out, or at least get near enough to transfer the patient if a Newcastle ambulance came up to meet them. Marc might not be able to survive the vibrations of a high-speed cross-country race for more than 100 miles, but then he might also have a heart attack here at the airport. There was no alternative. This was his only chance.

'Okay, son, here we go,' said Norrie aloud, looking back at the ambulance through the rear window of the police car as it led the way out of the airport. 'Hold on tight!'

SIX

MARTIN

'You're shivering, we've got to go home to get you sorted,' said Sue's mother as they left Grantham Hospital in the early hours of that Wednesday morning, having seen the ambulance carrying Martin set off for Nottingham at high speed. Shock was setting in. Sue only had on a T-shirt and jeans and the dawn was chilly. The ambulance driver had told her father that it was pointless to try and follow behind, so they went back briefly to her house first and Sue found some warmer clothes. Rocky, their grizzled old Border Collie, was baffled by all these people turning up in his kitchen so early, booting him out into the garden to do his business.

'Come on, old boy, we don't know when we'll be home again,' said Len, helping the dog out of the door with the side of his foot, but Rocky didn't get it. He did what he had to do, then came straight back in and flopped back into bed.

'Where can we put a key?'

Len was thinking ahead. They put it under a pot in the shed and left that door unlocked. 'I'll phone your friend later and get her to take the dog,' said Joan. She would also phone Sue's office and tell them what was happening, assuming control of that side of things to help out her daughter.

Sue was barely there. She was thinking of Martin and the bleed on his brain, whatever that meant. The hospital staff had not said much more. She was thinking about brain damage. She was thinking about therapy and what that meant and what it cost and whether she would have to give up work to care for him at least for a while and whether their house would have to be adapted in some way, until he was better. He was alive, at least. Whatever happened, he was still her boy. His ambulance would have arrived in Nottingham by now. Their journey took an hour, with her father driving painfully slowly and Sue got exasperated, believing the doctors could not operate on her son without her permission.

'Go faster, Dad. Go faster! I haven't signed anything, they can't take him into theatre without my signature as a parent, you've got to speed up here.' But Len wouldn't go faster, for fear of crashing. They had to follow a map, they didn't know where they were going and when they got to the vast Queen's Medical Centre – the biggest hospital in the country at the time, with more than a thousand beds – and were eventually able to find the intensive care unit, the night sister had not heard of a Martin Burton. 'Sorry, we don't have anyone of that name. Where have you come from again? No, we've not had any patients from Grantham here and I don't think we're expecting any.'

Sue panicked then, but the sister looked at her again. 'Hang on, what age is your son? Sixteen? You want PICU then, he might be there.'

A young male nurse who didn't look much older than Martin himself explained in a kindly voice that the P was for paediatric, for kids. She knew that, of course, but her head wasn't working properly. He walked them there, ten minutes away through the labyrinth of the hospital, up to the fifth floor in the lift and through corridors that confused and this time the answer was yes, they had Martin. 'Or we will have, he's just coming back from theatre.' So they were already operating without asking, thought Sue. He must be in a really bad way. Her stomach twisted tighter. There was tea or coffee in the family room, but she didn't want either. There were tissues, but she was past tears. There was nothing to do now but wait.

* * *

The hammering on the door startled Nigel Burton as he lay awake in a bed far from home, on the other side of the Atlantic and on the far side of America.

'Yes? What?'

It was still Tuesday night there, eight hours behind Nottingham.

'Chief Tech Burton?'

The big, bulky Sergeant Supplier with a grim look on his face clearly hadn't come to drag Nigel out on the town. 'I've had a call from the guard room at Cottesmore.'

They worked at the same base in England but were staying in apartments on Las Vegas Boulevard for 'Red Flag', an advanced aerial combat exercise in the skies above Nevada. Red versus Blue with live bombs, the RAF on the side of the good guys in raids and dogfights across hundreds of miles, training for serious combat. Nigel was the liaison between the pilots and the ground crews that kept the planes flying. The Sergeant Supplier at his door saw to the spare parts, but they knew each other only by sight. Whatever this was about, couldn't it wait? Nigel had been up at half past four that morning and out to Nellis Air Force Base on the edge of town to get the first wave of Harrier Jump Jets away. He'd turned down a trip to the Strip with the lads for an early night, but clearly wasn't going to get it.

'One of your sons has collapsed and they'd like you to phone home.'

Nigel had served his country in wartime, and this carefully spoken man with a dark moustache and close-cropped, thinning hair was known and admired for being cool under pressure. He was trained to put other worries to the back of his mind and focus on the task in hand. This news was nothing he could not handle, although somebody at home had obviously thought it was serious enough to ring the helpline for forces families, which was how he had been traced and told. He didn't expect it was Christopher who was poorly, Martin was the one who was always tripping over his own feet. He once fell off his skateboard and they took him to hospital then, but it all worked out okay. Fully expecting to be told that the crisis had passed, he rang home. There was no answer. Len and Joan did not reply to the phone at their house either. Nigel rang his own father, who knew nothing.

'It's very early here.'

Nigel told the sergeant he was not too worried.

'These things happen. It will be fine, I'm sure.'

They sat in the apartment kitchen while Nigel kept trying to call home without success, but the next person he spoke to was a squadron leader calling from RAF Innsworth in Gloucestershire, the management centre for the RAF, who said he had been tasked with getting Nigel home. That was alarming. They didn't pay for a commercial ticket back to the UK without a good, urgent reason, particularly if you were the only person in your unit who could do your job during an important exercise.

'All I can tell you at the moment is that Martin has collapsed and it is serious. The earliest I can get you out of Vegas is 07.45 hours tomorrow morning. You will have to stop over in Pittsburgh for three hours, then catch the Gatwick flight from there. It's the quickest way. We'll have a car at the airport to take you to Nottingham. We'll get you to your son as fast as we can.'

Fine, thought Nigel, as he started to pack his two kit bags, alone again in his room, but why the massive rush? There must be something he was not being told. Something terrible.

SEVEN

MARC

The police car rode the hills like a speedboat on the waves. Pushed back into his seat by the force of it all, Norrie felt sick to the stomach and gripped the hand rest with fright. He didn't dare look at the speedometer. They were plunging into deep space, with the blackness wrapping back around them in the rearview mirror. The ambulance was just about in their slipstream, but suddenly they were slowing down.

'What's up? What are we doing?'

'This is England. We have to stop.'

The ambulance passed by at speed as they pulled over and Norrie was alarmed. 'You're not gonna let them leave me behind?'

'No way. See?'

Another police car sat in the lay-by ahead, this time with the markings of the Northumberland Police.

'Come on, Norrie, let's get you swapped,' the officer said as he grabbed the spare oxygen bottles out from the back seat, letting in a rush of cold air. Norrie quickly tried to climb in the back of the next car but the door wouldn't open.

'No, Jock,' said the driver, an Englishman on his own in the car. 'You sit up front with me.' Norrie would have got cross if anyone else had called him Jock, but he wasn't going to argue with the only man who could get him to his son. The ambulance had disappeared over the hill but the driver saw him looking after it and grinned. 'Don't worry, Jock, we'll catch them.'

What happened next was a shock, says Norrie. 'I swear it was like being in a plane. We nearly took off. I thought, "My god, he's bombing it!"'

They had been going fast before, north of the border, but this was something else and it made Norrie laugh. He was getting hysterical with the grief, the stress and the fear, but he was elated, too – they were doing something for Marc at last, going somewhere fast, getting the best help they could. At least they were trying, all these people – the doctors, the nurses, the paramedics, the cops – all on his son's side. They were hurtling through the dark again now, but he knew they were heading down through the open country of the Northumberland National Park. 'I could see the ambulance far off in front, but there were hills, so the tail lights would pop up red in the distance then they'd disappear.'

The lights started to get closer but Norrie suddenly began to feel really sick.

'Are you all right?' The driver must have heard him groan.

'Not really. Can I have a cigarette, to settle my nerves?'

'What? No, pal. You're in a police car!' The driver was concentrating on the road but he must have thought about his passenger and how there would be nobody else to clear up the sick, because he changed his mind. 'Special circumstances? All right, you can.'

The window next to Norrie opened just a crack and the wind raged in his ear, but it was clear what he was expected to try and do. So he lit his fag, took a drag, craned his neck and tried to blow smoke out of the window. They were going at more than 100 miles an hour. The wind blew the smoke back in his eyes and the ash in his mouth, all over his face. The driver laughed. 'Nice one, Jock.'

Norrie laughed too, high on adrenaline. It felt like seconds before they were in among houses and street lights again and the shop signs suggested they were on the edge of Newcastle, where two other patrol cars joined them. 'My mates are going to play tag,' said the driver, meaning that one car would race ahead and block off the road for the ambulance to pass through, then the other would accelerate away to the next junction to do the same. 'I felt like I was in a movie,' says Norrie, who had never seen such driving. Jock or not, he was grateful. 'I couldn't thank those guys enough for what they did that night.'

Still, when they got to the Freeman Hospital in Newcastle the distractions of the drive fell away and he was hit again by the full force of what was happening to his son. Norrie expected to walk into the hospital and be told that Marc was dead, but there was nobody there to meet them. The English policeman led the way up the stairs, but as they were going up he saw the doctor and nurses who had ridden with the ambulance coming towards him. There were four women and the older man, the medic he recognised from before, looking exhausted now. The man's face was wet with tears, and Norrie felt a rush of despair, as he realised what that meant. It had all been in vain. Marc had not made it.

But as they passed on the stairs, the man reached out and put a hand on his shoulder. Norrie braced himself.

'Your son's a fighter. He's still with us in there …'

EIGHT

MARTIN

When his phone rang at home at five-thirty on the Wednesday morning, the doctor who would take charge of Martin's care at Nottingham was already awake. Harish Vyas was an early riser, no matter what time he had gone to bed. He answered quickly, so as not to disturb his wife and four sons asleep in their home in a village to the north of Nottingham. This was his sanctuary, the place to which he came home after the long days and nights that so often ran together on the ward, but he was always ready to return to the hospital at a moment's notice. If there was one thing you could say about this comfortably built man in his mid-fifties with his swept-back hair and greying brush of a moustache, it was that he really cared. Other doctors knew how to detach themselves from work and walk away at the end of the day for their own survival, but not him. 'I am an emotional being, that is who I am. I have chosen not to fight it. I cannot help becoming involved.'

Dr Vyas was in charge of the children's intensive care unit at the Queen's Medical Centre in Nottingham, with a dozen patients at any one time, and he felt for every family. He knew the names of mothers, fathers, sisters and brothers, grandparents and carers and sometimes even pets, and once he was involved in an urgent case he found it hard to leave the hospital. 'I could go on without much sleep for five or six days at a time, easily. This is really personal. You talk to the family, you stick with them and you don't want the baton to be passed on to somebody new, for their sake.'

The unit required hard work and very long hours and needed a certain stamina and commitment. Working together in this environment produced phenomenal loyalty among the doctors and nurses. The ward sister knew he would come. She had only called because it was really important.

'A young man of sixteen is coming to us from Grantham with significant neurological features. It could be a bleed on the brain. He is going straight for a scan and then to theatre.'

Sixteen years old. The same age as one of his own sons, sleeping safe. Harish Vyas thought of that as he drove up the hill away from his village and down to the hospital, through the dawn. It was only three hours since Martin's collapse. 'The brains of children are very different from adult brains,' the doctor says now, looking back at that moment. 'They have such amazing resilience. I saw a young girl who was brought in after a wardrobe fell on her and she was crushed. She had multiple fractures and a bleed in the brain. When she came to the emergency department, she was squirting blood from her nose. After surgery, I brought her over to our unit and ventilated her and, to cut a long story short, she is now back to normal. So children do surprise me. But Martin was, perhaps, a bit old.'

The brain is a fragile thing. Squishy to the touch, it looks like half a ball of fatty, uncooked sausagemeat bound up in clingfilm. It weighs three pounds, the same as a big bag of flour, but doesn't feel that heavy in your head because it actually floats around, suspended in a salty fluid. This odd lump of white and grey matter is – by some miracle – the place where our thoughts and feelings occur, but it is also the beginning of the central nervous system that controls every part of the body. From here, the orders go out to make the heart beat, the lungs breathe, the tongue taste, the eyes see, the nose smell, the ears hear and the skin feel.

All this is done by 100 billion nerve cells which need oxygen to survive and thrive. Without it they begin to die, and that can cause headaches and seizures, take away the ability to speak, paralyse the body or ultimately kill. That vital oxygen comes from the lungs and is carried in the blood pumped up by the heart, through the neck to the head, where the arteries wrap themselves around the brain like an intricate cradle of incredibly thin fingers. At the tip of each finger is a patch where the blood gives up the oxygen and takes away carbon dioxide, turning purple in the process. Then the old purple blood is carried away by a spidery network of veins, back down the neck to be pumped again through the heart and lungs and refreshed.

Sometimes, disastrously, the arteries or the veins just burst. The blood floods between the brain and the skull. This bleeding is what the emergency neurosurgeons at the Queen's Medical Centre in Nottingham could see had happened to Martin as they examined his brain scan in the early hours of Wednesday morning, although they could not yet be sure of the cause. It might have been the result of a head injury, like the one suffered by the little girl Dr Vyas was talking about – perhaps if he had fallen out of bed in the night. Or possibly a condition called Arteriovenous Malformation, a tiny tangling of the veins and arteries that could have been secretly lurking in his head for years, even since birth. They did know that he was bleeding heavily – catastrophically, in medical terms – and the blood had formed a clot that was pressing down on his soft brain like a butcher's thumb.

There was no time to waste: it was three or four hours since Sue had seen Martin collapse and the surgeons suspected his condition was getting worse by the minute. They could not wait for his mother to arrive at the hospital, to explain to her what the scan had shown and to ask her permission to act, so they took Martin straight to theatre. There, the surgeons drilled a hole in the skull to let some blood flow out and to relieve the pressure and they sucked out the clot as best they could, hoping that the brain would stop swelling. If it did not then it would continue to get bigger, pressing upwards against the inside of his skull and downwards through the brain stem, the three-inch stalk that connects the brain with the spinal cord and controls vital functions like the heart rate, breathing and sleeping. Drugs were used to paralyse Martin and keep him from writhing about, because any movement was going to make things worse. A very high dose of morphine stopped him feeling any pain. He was being kept in a coma for his own good.

* * *

When Martin came back from surgery, he was put on his own in the room nearest the entrance to the intensive care unit. Reserved for the most serious cases, Cub 2, as the little sign with a cheeky monkey said, was away from the rest of the ward so that fretting mums and dads whose sons or daughters were close to death did not have to see the other children, who were mostly getting better, and the other children and their families did not have to see them. Sue and her parents were shown a kettle and supplies in the family room for hot drinks and a microwave to heat up food if they felt like eating, which they did not. They sat on two sofas staring at the television without seeing anything, minds hazy with the interference of anxiety and fear. Harish Vyas could see the distress on their faces as they stood up when he entered the room.

'Would you like to sit down?'

He introduced himself and offered tea and biscuits, knowing that even in moments of high anxiety, people often have an urge to sip a drink and perhaps taste something sweet. There were no takers this time.

'Can I ask what else you have been told?'

Something about a bleed on the brain said Sue, and the doctor agreed.

'The most likely event is that the blood vessels in his brain have burst. The extra blood has caused pressure to build up inside his head.'

A registrar who had come up from the operating theatre two floors below explained what had been done in surgery, and that sickened Sue. Then Dr Vyas took over again, gently but firmly. They needed to see how he would settle down and do some more tests before they could be sure what had caused this and what might happen next.

'If I can just prepare you a little, Martin is still very poorly. He has a tube in his mouth and there are various lines into him. These things are all part and parcel of his treatment here. You will notice that he isn't moving, this is because of the drugs we give him to prevent any more problems. Would you like to see Martin now?'

If Martin had been awake he could have looked out of the window and seen the early morning sky. The pale blue curtains were drawn back, offering a grim view of air conditioning units and the flat top of the next hospital block, but the sky was out there too, distant and hopeful. But this handsome young lad could see nothing with his eyes closed and there was no prospect of them opening soon, not even when his mother entered the room. He lay flat on his back on a white iron bed with his head in a support block and a white, corrugated plastic pipe going into his mouth and down into his oesophagus for the ventilator, feeding air into his lungs to help them work. The monitors behind him showed a series of squiggly lines, changing all the time: blood pressure, heart rate, oxygen levels and the reading from a gauge on the end of a hairline wire going into his head. Half a dozen pumps sent drugs into his body through a single feed in the groin – 'the hosepipe', as the staff called it when there was nobody else around. Martin wasn't moving, except for the rise and fall of his chest.

'You can touch him,' said the nurse gently, feeling Sue hold back. 'It's okay.'

She went closer then, feeling the warmth rising from his body, or maybe it was the warm air under the blanket, but it was suddenly hot in that room, stiflingly so, prickling her neck. Sue kissed the tips of her fingers and placed them on his forehead, pushing them through his hair.

'Oh, Martin. What are we going to do with you?'

'Call for you,' said a nurse at the door and Sue went to the desk confused, but it was Nigel on a crackly line from Las Vegas, sounding far away. She was just about able to hold it together and describe the situation, as much as she had been told and could remember, until she had to tell him the condition Martin was in, right there and then. 'He's got a bleed in the brain. We don't know what the outcome is going to be, we don't know …' Her voice cracked and Nigel also struggled not to lose control. 'I'll get there as soon as I can.'

Sue put the phone down and turned back to the reality of the ward, momentarily thrown, before being overcome by a rush of concern for her other son Christopher, aged twenty, who had arrived with his girl-friend, Ashley. 'I was split between the two boys, divided between thinking about Martin on life support and worrying how Chris was coping with it. Christopher was very angry that he couldn't do anything to protect Martin. He was very angry that Nigel wasn't there. I think he felt he had to be the man. He kept having to go out to go off for a walk. I think he was letting himself vent that anger by storm-ing around outside the hospital, rather than actually sitting with Martin and showing his emotions.'

'Ashley stayed with him the whole time. If he moved, she moved. I was aware that he was a very angry young man right then and I wanted her to not have to deal with that, so I said to Ashley, "If he gets more angry and you need anybody, just fetch my dad."'

Back at Martin's bedside, for the sake of something to say to the young nurse in blue who was moving around her son, Sue began to ask questions. 'What will happen now? If everything is for the best, how long do you think it might be before Martin could come home? We'll do whatever is necessary for him, obviously …'

The way the nurse responded made Sue realise with a lurch that she might be getting this wrong. Everything she was fearing and dreading might actually be too much to hope for.

'We'll wake him up slowly,' the nurse said cautiously. 'Then we'll wait and see.'

NINE

MARC

Somewhere south of the border, Linda was struggling too. She was in her own car with Leasa travelling to Newcastle when she felt her tongue swell up inside her mouth until she couldn't talk. Her lips ballooned and her eyes became raw, weeping like they were full of grit.

'Oh my God, what's happened to you?'

The nurse who met them at the Freeman was shocked and treated Linda straight away. She had been given a couple of pills for a headache by a paramedic up in Scotland and was suffering an allergic reaction. The symptoms were dramatic but they would pass away with the right drugs. Linda was weak though and she needed to be put under observation. A porter pushed her to a ward in a wheelchair.

'I was sedated and they kept me in overnight, with large doses of antihistamines. That was a really bad start, I just wanted to be with my boy.'

Norrie was already at the hospital and couldn't believe it when Leasa found him and told him. 'Seriously, that could only happen to Linda. Unbelievable.'

She was going to be okay though, it was just a bit of a drama. Leasa shook her head and made a joke about how her emotional mum was the centre of attention, even now.

'There's no show without Punch.'

Linda was brought up in a village to the west of Glasgow, a country girl who fell for the first handsome boy she met at her first proper disco in the local town, when she was just seventeen. His name was Norman but everybody called him Norrie.

'We just clicked right away.'

He was short and sharp, gregarious and funny, but not one for candlelight or flowers. 'There was no romance. Never.'

Within six months, to the horror of both their parents, Linda was pregnant. Norrie proposed. Sort of. 'My granny and my father think we should get married because you're pregnant. They'll pay for the register office in Johnstone, which is £36.'

'There were no violins,' says Linda. 'We were too young. I'd hardly been out with any boys. I hadn't lived my life. I hadn't even been to the dancing before and I had to stop anyway because of the baby.'

Linda was seven months pregnant on the day they got married in 1981. The only witnesses were a couple who were their friends. 'We had a meal. Then I went home and made my bed, cos I was knackered.'

Leasa was the first child to arrive, a beautiful, very calm baby, who would grow up to become a strong young woman. Then came Darren and Ryan, both proper lads, destined to be a soldier and a professional footballer. Marc was next, the sparky little lad they all doted on and called over for cuddles. 'Marc gave me the least bother. He was never ill and he never got in trouble at school. If there was a cat or a dog in the house it would go straight to Marc, he had a really good soul. Very laid-back and never complained about nothing. A wonderful brother to his sister Leasa, really dedicated to his brothers and his friends. A very caring son.' He was very shy, though. 'If anyone spoke to Marc he went scarlet.'

Linda was proud of her kids, but seeing them grow up and get on with their own lives was a struggle for her sometimes. They needed her less and less. Marc became her ally against the passing of time. He was the one she could still hold close and keep safe, until a fifth child came along. 'I was pregnant for the whole of the Eighties,' she says with a laugh. 'I kept trying for another girl. I was like, "Norrie, one more time, please?" I never got her!'

The youngest, baby Daryl, was poorly with a hip disease for a while and had to be in a wheelchair at the age of four. 'That probably stopped me having any more kids. "I don't need a pram, I've got a wheelchair!"'

By then Marc was away running with a pack of cheeky lads from the same street, with a river to swim in, a waterfall to jump over and a wood for games. But when all her own boys were home indoors, the house was a riot. 'Darren was the funny, cocky one who made us all laugh. Ryan was the daddy who'd say: "I've got football in the morning, youse better stop making a noise." Marc was the peacekeeper, the negotiator. He'd say to his brothers, "What did you say that to Leasa for? You need to go and say sorry." What a wain.' Leasa was like a second mother. 'She's one of the best folk I know in the world. She's lost more than a brother. Leasa taught Marc to walk when she was five or six and he was just a baby.'

Once the kids didn't need her so much, Linda trained to follow her own mother Betty into the health service and started as a nursing assistant at the Royal Alexandra Hospital in 1991, working the twilight shift four times a week in the respiratory ward, doing everything a nurse would do except giving controlled drugs. That meant looking after people who were on diamorphine at the end of their life, as they succumbed to lung cancer. 'I was very good at that, giving people respect in those times. Nothing prepares you for seeing your first dead body though, or having relatives screaming in your face. Or patients that have got cancer in their brain and they're violent with you.'

She soon saw a person die. 'A wee old man called Robert. Nobody was sitting with him, so I did. After that, I couldn't count how many people I was with in their last moments. We would strip the bed and get the person decent for their relatives to see. We'd get a vase – no red and white flowers in the same vase, it was bad luck – clear the room of any medical equipment, dim the lights and have it looking nice. Open the window to let the person's soul out.'

She means that. It was superstition, but sincere. There were leaflets with advice for the family and she would ask if they wanted her to call anyone. 'We had good china, so I would get a tray and set it up for the relatives, get some good hankies, give them a wee pat and listen, if they wanted to talk about their loved one.' She really cared for those people. 'I loved my job.'

Norrie was working hard as a roofer and if he had come straight home at night she would have been at the hospital anyway, so he tended not to. 'He was only a young guy back then, so he was at snooker one night, football the next, the pub another and golfing the next. I thought, "D'ye know what? I earn good money. I manage fine. I don't need a drunk man coming in at night, out ye go!"' They split up in 1996 but are still friends to this day. 'I could phone him for anything and Norrie would do it for me. Nobody will ever love or care for our kids the way he does.'

The new machine at Newcastle saved Marc's life, at least for that first day. It took old blood out of a tube in his leg, warmed it and removed the carbon dioxide, refreshed the blood with oxygen and pumped it back into him, taking over from his heart to manage his whole circulation. His chances of getting through the next day and night rose above one per cent now, but he was still as sick as any living patient the nurses in Newcastle had ever seen. And there was a serious catch. The longer he was on the machine, the greater the chance of an infection that could kill him anyway.

A heart had to be found from somewhere fast.

TEN

MARTIN

Nigel called the hospital at Nottingham again just before he boarded the plane to Pittsburgh very early on Wednesday morning in Las Vegas and he was answered by his mother-in-law, Joan. It was now the Wednesday afternoon in England, about twelve hours after Martin's collapse. Joan said nothing had changed since the last call.

'My wife wasn't talking to me, she didn't want to leave Martin to come to the phone, so I knew it was very serious. I was starting to get the feeling that this was not going to be a good outcome.'

Nobody spoke to him on the four-hour flight across Middle America, as they passed from west to east over the deserts of Utah, the mountains of Colorado, the plains of Kansas, then Illinois, Indiana, Ohio and finally, Pennsylvania. The couple in the next two seats slept all the way, so the introverted Englishman was left alone, thousands of miles from home and five miles up in the air, with dark feelings of guilt. 'I was in the wrong place. I couldn't have been further away from him if I had tried. It felt wrong. I was thinking about the times when the boys said I was never home.'

He loved them both dearly, more than they knew. His way of coping with all the time abroad was to crack on with work and try not to mope, but he gave them his full attention when he was home. Now the feelings that he usually tried to keep in check began to rise and threatened to flood over him. The wait at Pittsburgh International Airport was three hours. Nigel found a payphone and called the hospital straight after arrival and got through to Joan again, who said the same as before. He put the phone down, walked through the crowds to the departure lounge and found a seat in a corner. 'That's when it really hit me: I was going home to say goodbye and switch the life support machine off. They needed my authority. I put my coat over my head and just wept and wept, because I knew I had lost my son.'

The thought was overwhelming, even though he had no real confirmation. This was just a hunch but it was a powerful one and it broke him. Fellow passengers of all ages were all around but Nigel felt completely on his own as he hid inside his coat, doubled over, sobbing and sobbing, rocking back and forth. 'I'm amazed nobody from security came over to say, "Why are you acting like this?" Nobody came to me or spoke to me. Nobody did anything. I would not wish that journey on anybody.'

Deep in his sorrow, Nigel went back over his last conversation with Martin on the phone again and again. 'I was sorry the last thing I had done was to deny him a gift. There was no sign of anything being wrong before I left. Did we miss something? Was there something more we could have done? It was just grief, sodden grief that I had lost my son and there was nothing I could do about it.'

Nobody had actually told him Martin was dead or even about to die. 'I was just assuming. There was a little nugget of hope that I was wrong but I don't think I honestly believed that. I felt like I just wanted to sit there and not do anything else, just put my head in my hands and weep and cry, but I couldn't, I had to get back. I wanted to be there for Sue and for my sons.'

His service training kicked in. Nigel found composure enough to board the aircraft. 'I just controlled myself because I knew that if I wasn't careful I wouldn't get on the plane, and that was the last thing I wanted. I managed to smile at the lady on the gate, hand her my boarding pass, go through and sit at my seat and then collapse again, because I could do that now, nobody was watching me. I could go back into my own little world.'

The man in the next seat chatted briefly, but they both fell silent after take-off. The screens came down and the movie started: *Bulletproof Monk*, an action comedy starring Chow Yun-Fat, which opens with a fight on a rope bridge, over a chasm. A young Buddhist completes his training with a master, who tells him this moment is: 'The end of my destiny, and the beginning of yours'. Nigel couldn't bear it.

'I took off the headphones and just sat there thinking about all that Martin was losing: his future, his aspirations, his wife to come maybe and his kids, there's just a huge hole that suddenly appears and you wonder how you will ever fill it. How could a pain like that ever get better?'

As his father was flying home, Martin was put through another CT scan. He had now been at Nottingham's Queen's Medical Centre for more than twelve hours. The results confirmed what Harish Vyas already suspected: there was no chance of recovery. The brain stem controlling his heart rate, breathing and other vital functions of the body had been crushed by the swelling brain and destroyed. Without it, Martin had no hope of surviving on his own. The consultant called for a colleague to give a second opinion and together they carried out a series of tests required by law in a situation like this, making sure that Martin did not react when they squirted cold air into his eyes or cold water into his ears. They watched as the ventilator was turned off for a short while, to see if Martin would somehow breathe on his own. He didn't, says Harish Vyas.

'The results of all the tests combined together indicated that the brain stem had effectively stopped functioning. In other words, Martin was brain dead.'

American law says all the functions of the brain have to stop before a person can be considered to have passed away, but in Britain it is enough to say that the brain stem no longer works. Some people disagree, but the law is clear and so is the doctor. Martin was never going to breathe on his own or wake up, it was impossible. His life was over.

'However he looked, lying there in the bed, there was no doubt that he was dead.'

Sue still thought they were trying to rescue her son and save him from serious brain damage, but all that was about to change when Harish Vyas came to see the family.

'I'm really sorry, but the extent of Martin's bleed is just so great that there is nothing we can do for him.'

After a moment of shocked silence, the raw reactions broke through. Sue's body shook, then the floodgates inside her burst and she shuddered and snarled and howled. The hurt was real. Sharp, physical, hard. Every nerve screaming. Len reached for Joan's hand. Christopher got angry, and Ashley held on to him. Dr Vyas tried to carry on explaining but he had lost them. Sue wasn't listening. 'I had acknowledged that Martin was going to be brain-damaged, that he could be at any level from a vegetative state upwards, but I had not even considered that he was not going to make it. It hit me like a hammer in the face, absolutely full on. I was being told that my child was going to die. Nothing else went in for a while.'

Harish Vyas could see she was hurting but he kept talking, quietly and carefully, offering what little reassurance he could by saying that Martin had probably been brain dead when the ambulance crew arrived.

'Martin has died peacefully, there was never any pain.'

Sue thought of her son standing in the doorway before he fell, unable to see her. She had read that hearing was the last of the senses to be lost when someone was dying. Her voice would have been the last thing he heard, calling his name.

Dr Vyas now had to ask a very delicate question. Perhaps the most difficult question a doctor can ask a mother when he has just told her there is no hope for her child.

'Have you considered organ donation?'

The timing was brutal but the doctor was absolutely convinced he was doing the right thing. 'There is never a good time to talk about this. Waiting half an hour was not going to make any difference.' Putting the question immediately meant the mother could answer before she was swept away by a tsunami of grief. Martin's lungs, liver, kidney and heart could save or extend lives. His corneas could help the blind see. 'There is a sense of urgency. If we don't move early, the organs deteriorate.'

Looking back, Sue agrees with what he did. 'You go into shock when you've been given this terrible, devastating news and you just collapse inside but then you've got to decide quite quickly. I now understand that it has to be quick. I was still *compos mentis*, before the emotions of what was happening began to sink in. I don't know whether two or three hours later I would have felt the same or even been able to answer. I would have gone to pieces and been so grief-stricken, I wouldn't have wanted anyone to touch him.'

As it was, she gave her answer without hesitation. 'Yes,' she said. 'Do it.'

'Nigel and I were already on the organ donor register, it was something we had talked about as a couple and agreed on. I would not have been able to put this into words at the time, but deep down, even then, I was looking for something positive to come out of this tragedy. Martin was young, he was a very healthy boy who had never had any time off school because of illness. No part of his body was damaged in any way, except his brain. Even at that point, I could see that it would have been sacrilege to have lost all of those healthy young organs and buried them with him.'

Sue paused for a moment in the hospital to ask her son Christopher his opinion and he agreed. 'In the midst of all that grief there was a clarity of thinking. I never ever had any second thoughts. I never, ever saw transplantation as a violation of Martin's body. I truly wanted to save some other family from going through the nightmare we were going through.'

The nurses were already working hard to keep Martin stable that Wednesday afternoon, trying to keep him going so that his dad, who was racing there from five thousand miles away, could have a few moments alone with him to say goodbye before the life support machine was turned off. They also wanted his body parts to be in the best possible condition. That was the harsh reality of it.

'Looking after children who are brain dead is a very complex problem. Once the brain stem dies there is an outpouring of chemicals that makes intensive care very difficult,' says Harish Vyas. Hormones flood the body and the organs begin to fail without the brain to tell them what to do. The lungs fill up with fluid. The blood pressure goes haywire without the signals to keep it under control and the circulation begins to slow and stop. The kidneys start to pour out urine. All this has to be stopped or overcome with drugs. Martin also had to be turned over often, to prevent his skin breaking down.

Meanwhile, his age, weight and blood type were sent urgently to the office running the NHS Organ Donation Register down in Bristol and samples were taken for blood- and tissue-matching tests. Specialist surgical units were put on stand-by to take his organs the next day. And all the while, says Harish Vyas, the nurses acted as if he was alive. 'Martin was nursed as if he was a patient who was on the way to recovery. We looked after his skin care, his mouth care and all the other aspects of nursing were carried on as normal. The nurses talked to him, continually. It is our normal practise to make sure we talk to our children and this was not absent in Martin's case.'

The consultant's wife brought in a razor and a change of clothes and he took a shower. He wouldn't go home until this was over. 'We didn't usually lose our patients like this. I couldn't just walk away.'

Sue sat with Martin and felt the staff work around her and was touched by their kindness. 'They were doing all this to someone they knew was brain dead.'

They put a heated airbed under Martin's body to keep him warm. A physio came every couple of hours to manipulate his chest and stop mucus building up on his lungs. A friend who had come to sit with Sue pointed out how young and pretty the nurse was. 'Martin would have liked her.'

They both sort of laughed. There was a curious relief in that.

The rest of the ward was still functioning too, with the lights down low. 'I heard them turn a child away that night because they had a bed but not enough staff. I found that quite hard to come to terms with, when I knew Martin was dying.'

Sue could not put her arms around him, though.

'That was the hardest thing. All I wanted was to hold him, touch him, whatever, but I wasn't able to do that because he was wired up and there were nurses surrounding him as if he was a patient they were fighting to keep alive. If we had not agreed to donation, then the machines would have been turned off and all the wires taken out and I don't think he would have lived for very long. He was too big to put on my knee, but at least then I could have held him.'

At least she could have let him go like that, bound up in her arms until the end. It just wasn't possible, though. And she did have extra hours to say goodbye, as Wednesday afternoon became the evening and the night. They were waiting for Nigel to come and say goodbye to his son, but the time was also needed to let other hospitals know the organs were coming and to assemble the surgical teams that could remove them. 'I couldn't leave Martin's side. I knew that I hadn't got very long. You can stay awake for a couple of days if you have to and I knew that time was limited so I just wanted to spend it with him, even if I was just looking at him.'

Sue spent her last night with her youngest son sitting in a hospital armchair by his bedside. Not knowing what else to do, she started to talk about the good times they'd shared together, hoping he could hear her now even though she knew deep down that he could not. She talked about the caravan they used to have when he was a little boy and their holidays. The time they went to Cyprus and he learned to swim. 'You lived in the pool all week. You went on holiday with armbands and you came back without them, we left them in the bin. That was lovely.'

Sue talked about their trip to Florida, which Martin had loved.

'Disneyland was awesome, remember? You were eleven.'

All this was her way of saying goodbye.

'That time was precious for me. Looking at him, wiping his eyes with a saline solution, giving his face a bit of a wash. The last things I could do as a mother. They were like last rites.'

She also kept reliving the moment Harish Vyas told her the bad news.

'The doctor was very clear that Martin was being kept alive by the machinery. They do want to make sure you totally understand that there is no hope. I knew that, of course, but now it began to really get inside my head and my heart. I began to realise that this was real, this was actually happening. I thought, "I gave birth to this child, how on earth do I live the rest of my life facing this loss?"'

This was the child she had carried in her womb and felt kicking inside her as she sung to him and whose life she had then released into the world. The baby who'd fed from her breast and whose nappy she had changed countless times. The little boy whose hands she held when he took his first steps and whose tears she wiped away when he fell. The infant she took to nursery for the first time, then to school, then to big school, giving him a quick kiss and ruffling his hair and turning away before he saw her tears. The growing lad who made her laugh, who made her cross when he was naughty but who could change her mood in a moment with a smile. The teenager who still called her 'Mummy' sometimes, when he wasn't thinking about it or when he thought nobody could hear. The boy who had sat with her on the sofa that last night at home, invading her space. She ached for that to happen again now, but it never would. Sue had been there for every moment of Martin's life and she was not going to leave him until the last, however much it was tearing her apart.

'As a mother, you want to care for your child right to the bitter end.'

ELEVEN

MARC

The McCays were given a flat to use in a block around the back of the hospital in Newcastle but they didn't want to leave the ward where Marc was being cared for. Linda was over her allergic reaction and back with her clan again by morning. 'Only two people were allowed in with Marc at a time, so we took turns and we slept upright in the chair or curled up on the two-seater sofa in the family room. I didn't want to take a sedative, I wanted my wits about me.'

They were quite a presence. There was another child on the same kind of equipment as Marc – the machine called an ECMO that Linda had no problem remembering because it was the only thing keeping her boy alive, taking the place of his heart. This child was also a boy from north of the border, as the Geordie nurses pointed out, trying to get a smile.

'The Scots have invaded.'

Linda quickly got to know the other boy's mother and his story. 'He was a fit and healthy wee boy, only three years old, who'd been running about the garden until a virus attacked his heart, same as Marc.' But no suitable heart had been found for him and the boy was now out of time. Linda saw how utterly, desperately silent the poor woman was in the moments after her little boy passed away, struck mute by her loss.

'His mum was destroyed. I was thinking, "This is what lies ahead."'

Marc needed a miracle, because that's what heart transplants are. Modern miracles of medicine, bravery and compassion. Healers and doctors have tried surgery for eight thousand years, but they did not dare to touch the heart until about a century ago. They either couldn't get to it without killing their patient or else they didn't want to go there at all, because the heart was considered too precious, the home of our deepest feelings and of the soul. Those old ideas echo in our words even now. Listen to your heart, the poets say. Follow your heart. The heart soars when your love is near and breaks when they leave. You wear your heart on your sleeve. You give your heart away. It's another word for instinct or emotion, the heart ruling the head, but it's also far more than that. Men and women have believed since the beginning of human history that the heart is special. The ancient Egyptians thought it was weighed against a feather in the afterlife, with a light heart as the sign of a good life. Others have said that the spirit or essence of a person sits in the heart or that God speaks to us there. Islamic scholars regard the heart as the most important part of the body; Christians talk about Jesus living in theirs. No wonder the heart was regarded as untouchable for so long. It's hard to get to anyway, hidden behind the ribcage, set deep in the body at the centre of everything. Only a rebel, a maverick or a wild dreamer would have dared to think of carrying out a transplant.

All of those words apply to Christiaan Barnard, a brash South African who stunned the world in 1967 by announcing that he had successfully taken the heart of a brain-dead young woman and put it in the failing body of a middle-aged man. The patient died of pneumonia after eighteen days, but by then the headlines had been made and Barnard was an international star. Brilliant, buccaneering surgeons like him went on trying to switch hearts when everyone around them thought it was mad or bad or just extremely dangerous to do. The patients kept dying too. But over the decades that followed, as the science improved, they began to live for longer and longer until the survival times were measured in years rather than days.

One of the nurses involved in the early days of heart transplants in Britain was a brisk, dynamic young woman called Lynne Holt, who would go on to lead the team looking after Marc McCay. Back in the early Eighties she saw hearts fail with dazzling, disturbing speed. 'You'd be talking to the patient, having a laugh, everything would be fine. Then you'd notice their blood pressure was slipping. They'd be dead six hours later, after acute rejection. The post-mortem would show they had a stone heart.'

The solution came – unlikely as it sounds – from an unusual bit of mould found growing in the soil on a high plateau in a remote part of Norway. A rare compound in the fungus was used to develop a new drug called Cyclosporine that could work to stop a new heart being rejected by the body but would not totally wipe out the ability to fight all infection. It was a life-saver and a game-changer for heart surgery in the Eighties.

'After that, you didn't see acute rejection any more. It transformed the whole process,' says Lynne, who joined the Freeman Hospital in Newcastle in 1986 as the first transplant co-ordinator anywhere in the country. She took charge of the whole process of find-ing the right organs for the right patients, getting them into theatre at the right time and supporting the families before and after surgery. Short, blonde and super-efficient, she wore a blue uniform with white trim. 'The uniform doesn't really portray the skill and the empathy, you know? A uniform is just the outer covering.'

By the time Marc McCay arrived in 2003, Lynne was leading a team of highly trained nurses available to help transplant patients and their families at any time, day or night. The hours were insane and Lynne didn't get to see her four young children as often as she wanted to. 'They were very used to Mummy not coming home at night and Daddy would read the story. I think you just feel very grateful when you go home eventually and you realise that their having a messy bedroom is not the end of the world.' Her feelings about being a working mum meant that when a child came to the hospital for a transplant it touched her deeply. 'That always stopped me in my tracks.'

When Marc arrived early on that Wednesday morning in late August, Lynne called an office in Bristol. His name was written in marker pen on a white board, at the top of a list of a dozen young patients needing transplants. His case was the most urgent, he was the closest to death. If a suitable heart became available anywhere in Britain, it would now be offered to him. There was still no guarantee it would come in time. The NHS was doing its best for Marc and the team caring for him was world class, but Lynne knew that even they might not be able to save him. 'Edinburgh had done an amazing job of keeping him alive but they had run out of options. We were his only hope.'

The day passed slowly for the McCays once Marc was in the intensive care unit, unconscious. They took turns to be with him but several of them were watching the television in the family room at the hospital, just for something to do, when the early evening news came on. There had been a crash on the A1, involving multiple cars. It was terrible, tragic. But somebody, quietly, said what they were all thinking. 'Could we get a heart out of that?'

Linda was horrified and said so, but then at the back of her mind, despite herself, she thought: 'Maybe. Yeah, maybe.'

'Some poor family will have to suffer for us, Mum,' said Leasa.

'Aye, I know, hen. I know. But listen, we have to be positive. Think about what it could mean for Marc. We've got to concentrate on that.' Linda felt she had to say that to her daughter, but she was also struggling. It was true, after all. They were waiting for someone to die.

Then it happened, suddenly. A nurse came and told them to brace themselves, because it looked like a heart would be available. A boy of the same age as Marc had passed away somewhere in England, she didn't know why. Tests were being made and details exchanged between hospitals but the early results looked good. The boy was otherwise fit and strong and had no medical problems, and he was the right blood type too. The nurses began to prepare Marc for surgery, in the knowledge that once the heart was removed from the donor it would have to be raced to the Freeman Hospital and inside Marc's chest within four hours to have any chance of working properly.

But nothing happened. The hours went by and Marc did not go to theatre, says Linda. 'We waited and waited for news until half-past three in the morning. Then they came and told us, bluntly – that's what they're like, but it's the best way to be – that it was not going to work.'

The doctor said it was impossible. 'I'm sorry, the young man was involved in a road accident, he went through the windscreen of the car. They could not have known this until they opened him up, but the heart was damaged. It can't be used.'

Linda wept again then, releasing all the hurt she had been holding inside all that day, dammed up by hope. She wept for the little lad and his family and for herself and her son too. 'I was devastated for this wee boy that had been killed but I was also devastated for Marc, who was still fighting for his life.'

Half a million people die in Britain every year, but that doesn't mean half a million hearts become available to save lives. Far from it. The number shrinks and shrinks when you take away those hearts that are diseased, destroyed or damaged at the point of death – like the one belonging to the boy in the car crash – or that are perfectly healthy but permission is refused. There's a big problem here, some say a national tragedy. Most people agree that organ donation is a good idea, but only a third of us carry a donor card.

There are all sorts of reasons why you might not have signed up for one yet. Maybe you've never given it much thought or you don't want to talk about death in case it comes too soon. Lots of people would say the same. Maybe the idea disgusts you: organ donation stirs up deep feelings. Maybe your religion says the body must be left intact for the afterlife or that bones and flesh will fly back together on the Day of Judgement. Even if you don't personally believe that any more, those ancient ideas are still so deep that they play on our minds and indeed our hearts. There it is again, the notion of the heart as the home of the soul, not to be messed with.

There is also the question of trust. Medical dramas like *Grey's Anatomy* sometimes suggest that doctors who want your organs for someone they really like will try a little less hard to save you. That doesn't happen in real life, but it is true that doctors are having a harder time trying to get us to trust them now, because of the medical scandals of recent years. All of this slashes the number of people who decide in advance that they will be organ donors – and even when they do, sometimes they are over-ruled after death. Mothers or fathers, sisters or brothers or lovers choose to ignore what they know the person wanted, because they cannot bear the thought of the body being divided and sent all over the place. They are distressed. It's a terrible time for them. Some are offended even to be asked, so they say no.

Incredibly, from a starting point of half a million deaths in Britain every year, only about 1,500 people are able and willing to give up their organs to save other lives. The supply of hearts almost vanishes when you add in the problem of finding one the right size for a child who needs saving, from a donor with the same blood type. Finally, the heart has to be taken out and rushed to the patient before it starts to deteriorate, which is very tricky. There were only seventeen heart transplants for children in the year Marc needed his. In the circumstances, it is extraordinary that there were any at all.

Linda was hurting, she got really wound up by people chatting or joking in the hospital canteen or corridors. 'I was so angry at the world, I wanted to say "What are you laughing at? What right do you have to laugh?" How dare they just get on with their lives? I actually felt quite cuckoo, but I was just reacting as a mum.'

Her mum and Marc's older brothers had arrived in Newcastle to join Leasa and Norrie and after the heart turned out not to be suitable they took turns by Marc's bedside so that poor agitated, exhausted Linda could try and get some rest. She was persuaded to take a sleeping tablet for her own good and had a bath up in the flat before managing to pass out in the bedroom in the early hours. But there was a loud bang as her son Ryan crashed into the place, breathless from having run across the whole hospital and up eight flights of stairs, in a hurry.

'Mum, wake up! There's a heart. You've got to come.'

She was muddled, drowsy, trying to get her clothes on but failing. Her hands wouldn't work properly, she kept banging into the walls as a result of the sleeping tablet. Ryan had to help her and take her arm, all the way down to the ward. Linda just wanted to sleep, to block it all out and forget, but she knew she had to wake up for Marc. Their excitement helped bring her round, it was infectious. 'This is it, here we go,' she said as the fog in her head cleared, and it was okay if they had to wait a couple of hours for the results of tests to see if this heart was the right one. She could wait; she could pray. As the day went on, she began to have faith that this one was going to work, this time.

Only it wasn't.

The donor was too old. There was too much risk of rejection. The arteries were diseased. Again, they only knew that when they cut him open. The doctor was sorry.

Linda didn't cry. She couldn't. There were no tears left.

She went in on her own to see her unconscious son, held his hand loosely around the clip and tube and told him again that she loved him, that she was not leaving until he was better, that she would always be there for him. He had to get better soon because his birthday was coming and there would be a big cake and a lot of laughs and everyone would be there, or they could go and eat out somewhere, wherever he wanted and it would be lovely, so he had to get better, okay?

Marc did not react. He was in deep, far away. The heart monitor pulsed. The ventilator wheezed. The blood machine carried on pumping, silently.

Linda felt someone standing behind her and turned to see one of Marc's doctors in the doorway, gesturing for her to come outside into the corridor.

'We've found another heart, Linda. A perfect match. This is the one.'

TWELVE

MARTIN

Nigel had been travelling for sixteen hours when the plane bringing him back to England touched down early on the Thursday morning. He had not been to bed for two days and he walked through the airport terminal with sudden flashes of longing, sleep-deprived day dreams of kissing his son on the forehead and having Martin wake up, sit up and say: 'What's the matter, Dad? Did you bring me a cuddly?' His head was in Vegas, it was at home in Grantham, it was in the park playing football with Martin, it was on the Gatwick escalator, it was in the hospital – it was in all these places at once.

There was a card with his name on it being held up by an elderly gentleman in the line at the arrivals gate. He put down his two enormous kit bags to shake the volunteer RAF driver by the hand. Then he heaved them onto his shoulders again for the walk to the car park.

The journey north to Nottingham took three hours, against the flow of the rush-hour traffic on the motorway. They spoke a little on the way, but not much. The driver was sensitive and careful not to intrude. Nigel mostly stared out of the window and watched the miles go by. He didn't know what to think or feel any more, he just wanted to be there. 'I would have hated not being with Martin when he died and not being able to say goodbye to my son. That would have been very painful.'

Nineteen hours after he had set off from Vegas, an exhausted Nigel finally hauled his bags into the paediatric intensive care unit. Before he could get to Sue, her mother stepped across his way.

'You know he's not going to make it, don't you?'

Joan was trying to protect her daughter. She wanted to be the one to tell him the bad news first, to take the pressure off Sue, who was in bits in the family room. Nigel was suddenly thrown by the realisation that she had not been entirely straight with him on the phone during his long journey. No, I didn't know that for sure, he thought, getting angry. His hunch had been right, but that was a father's instinct. 'You didn't tell me, but I've worked it out for myself, thank you!'

It wasn't her fault, he understood that later. Sue and Joan had both given him as little information as possible. Enough to make him set off for home, but not so much that he would break down in despair. Given what had happened in Pittsburgh anyway, maybe that was wise. Nigel had been awake for more than forty-eight hours straight when he went in to see his son.

'He was pink. He was warm. The only thing he had in his body that I could see was the breathing tube, but he looked like a sleeping Martin. There were no injuries, nothing to suggest the seriousness of the situation. Sue got up, tears streaming down her face, and put her arms around me. We hugged each other and cried. What else can you do?'

Nigel and Sue were left alone in the room now, just the two of them with their son Martin, for the first and only time. Sue felt enormous relief that she was no longer alone. Her parents, her son and his girlfriend had been great but Nigel was the one she needed. This was too much even for a Forces wife to cope with. It was difficult to know what to say, though. They held each other tight, but only briefly before they both turned back to look at Martin. The nurses continued to watch the monitors through the glass. Nigel was relieved to be there at last, but he was also numb.

'I just wanted to shake him and say, "Martin, wake up! Snap out of this!" But you know that's never going to happen. Then the nurse comes in again and starts doing things like checking his blood pressure and that brings the reality home.'

Sue told him quickly that she had agreed to organ donation.

'She knew my views. I said, "Yes, let's take some positives out of this very terrible, tragic situation. We are going to have to cope with his loss, irrespective of what decision we make, but let's try to make somebody else's life better today. Because our lives aren't going to be better."'

Sue had been thinking about it, too. 'We are going to have to face a life without our child and that is going to be hard, but there are other families out there that maybe won't have to sit where we are now, if we do this.'

She was sure Martin would have agreed with what they were about to do to him. 'He wanted to be a nurse, he was such a lovely boy who wanted to help people all the time and here's a way he could do that.'

There was paperwork to sign. A lot of it. The pair of them sat in a small, windowless, airless room on that Thursday morning with the hospital's transplant co-ordinator, yet more tea and a pile of forms. One each for the heart, lungs, liver, kidneys, pancreas and corneas. 'You have to authorise every organ. Each time you sign, you think about how this is a part of your child that is going to be taken and gifted to some-one else,' said Nigel.

They did not agree for the organs to be used in medical research. 'At the time it seemed a step too far, a little bit too much of a violation to have those organs used and chopped into little pieces and used for research,' says Sue. 'I would agree to it now, because I know that without research none of this could have happened, but at the time it was too much to deal with.'

By now, the word had gone out across the country that here was an unusually suitable donor boy with healthy organs. Matches were being made. Transplant cars were being booked to take the organs away from the hospital in Nottingham to wherever else they were needed. Planes too, as it turned out. Once his body was divided, the parts would be taken north and south, east and west, although the Burtons would not know to where. But for Nigel and Sue, that last Thursday afternoon was mostly spent watching as Martin's many friends came to say goodbye.

They arrived nervous and chatty but usually left in silence, says Sue. 'I made sure that myself or my mum met every one of them before they went into the room where Martin was, to make sure they knew what was happening, that he was actually dying.'

The language was difficult. He was not really dying: Martin's life was over, there was no more brain activity, he was legally dead, even if the rest of his body still looked perfectly normal and was still working, thanks to the life support machines.

'I wanted them to know that he would just look like Martin asleep in a hospital bed with some wires attached, he was not even covered in wounds or bandages and he did not look like a dead body. That was what they were afraid of. Everybody thinks that a dead body is going to be scary, don't they?'

The mother of one of the boys brought a carload over. Then a pretty, dark-haired girl from Sleaford called Michelle turned up with her friend, having come on the bus and the train. That was quite a trek.

'I'm Martin's girlfriend,' she said.

'Are you?'

Sue was shocked. Martin was not a boy who could keep a secret, she thought. If anything, he shared too much of his private thoughts and feelings with his mum, it could get a bit embarrassing, but this was something new and unexpected.

'Oh yeah,' said Michelle. 'He bought me a teddy.'

'Did he?'

'Yeah. I've bought him a St Christopher necklace, to go in his coffin.'

Sue and Nigel both struggled to take all this in,

although Michelle seemed like a very nice girl. 'She was lovely. We always wondered what kind of a girl he would bring home,' remembers his mother, who would later find pictures of her on Martin's computer at home. 'Obviously there was something quite strong going on between them but we didn't know, he didn't let on. Every time he saw kissing on the television he would be like, "Agh! Sloppy bits!" So the last thing we expected was for Martin to have a girlfriend, but it was a pleasant shock. One of the only amusing things to come out of that day.'

A nurse called Anna who seemed to have stayed on after her shift just to look after them pointed out with a smile how many young women had come to see him. 'We've had a string of teenage girls through here, haven't we?'

She brought a fresh cup of tea every time there were tears, says Sue. 'Anna was wonderful. I was water-logged with tea by the end of the day.'

Sue was worried that the doctors would come suddenly for Martin without warning, so she asked them to give her lots of notice. 'We knew we were going to leave him then. So when he left that room and we left that room, that would be the last time we would see our son breathing.'

She still could not think of him as dead, despite what she had said to all the kids.

'It's very hard to sit with someone who is pink and warm and not see them as alive. I was sitting there holding his hand, he was alive. In my mind, anyway.'

Sue was offered the chance to go with Martin, walking alongside his bed right to the door of the operating theatre, but she said no. She would say goodbye here, privately, in his room. The transplant co-ordinator from the hospital said kindly that she would accompany him instead and promised: 'We will treat him with as much care as if we were saving his life.'

As Thursday evening came, Sue was aware that time was running out. The nurses said Martin would be leaving at 8 pm. 'The last hour was probably the hardest. We had been through thirty-six hours of this at the hospital and although we agreed with what was happening, when it came up close it was much harder to cope with. I felt I could sit there forever with him. While I was sitting there, it wasn't the end.'

But it was the end. It had to be.

Harish Vyas was there to say so, personally. As the nurses were checking the monitors for one last time, the consultant met Nigel in the doorway to the room. 'Martin will be going to theatre for the removal of his organs very soon. I think we need to say goodbyes now.'

A nurse was beginning to work the translucent blue bellows of the ventilator by hand, as she would have to do all the way to the theatre. The bed was being turned now and Martin was coming towards them slowly, head first.

The consultant saw tears on Nigel's face, but then he felt a touch on his shoulder as they were both standing in the doorway and heard unexpected, tender words.

'Thank you. I didn't know you guys cared.'

Dr Vyas realised that he, too, was weeping.

'The day I stop caring is the day I pack my bags and leave this place. I am so sorry for your loss,' he told Martin's father. 'I wish we could have done more but there was nothing we could do. I am so sorry.'

The porters who had come to remove Martin on Thursday night paused out of respect for Sue, who was still bending over the body. She couldn't say goodbye. She just couldn't, even when her dad took her arm. 'We have to go now, love.'

'Susan, it's time,' Nigel said tenderly, using her full name, but there was almost a scuffle. 'We tried to get her out of the door of the unit and that was very hard. She just fought because she didn't want to leave her son, she found it extremely difficult to do that. We had to more or less force her out. She was in tears and we were all very emotional. You can understand that.'

Sue knew this was the moment to let go. She felt everyone around her watching. It was the sensible thing, but it was so hard. Too hard. 'I felt I was leaving him. I know now that he had been dead for at least twenty-four hours already, but that was the moment that I felt it was the end, for me. Not the day before. So it was excruciatingly difficult. I wanted to stay there. I wanted Martin to stay there, so I could be with him. To walk out of that hospital was the hardest thing in the world.'

There was no choice, though. It was just after 8 pm on Thursday 28 August. She held her child one last time, kissed his face and whispered in his ear.

'Sleep tight. We'll love you forever.'

THIRTEEN

MARTIN & MARC

They gathered outside the operating theatre in Nottingham as that Thursday night wore on: a dozen doctors and nurses, anaesthetists and surgeons in their green scrubs and gowns, waiting to take turns to retrieve the organs from the still-warm body of Martin Burton. His heart was still beating, his body was still working, with the assistance of drugs and machines, even though his brain was dead and his life was legally over. A single, long sweep of the scalpel from his throat to his waistline opened Martin up and the long process began. The heart would be removed first, but not until the early hours of the morning. A specialist team from the Papworth, the world-famous transplant hospital in Cambridge, had come across the country to take charge of this part of the operation. They could see from the colour of the heart and the way it was beating that this was a healthy organ, one that could save a life.

A heart like this is the size of a fist. It clenches – or beats – somewhere between sixty and a hundred and twenty times a minute, depending on how hard the body is having to work at the time. The clench happens when a chemical reaction in the blood creates a tiny pulse of natural electricity that causes the meaty muscle to contract, squeezing out the blood that has filled the hollow chambers inside the heart while it was relaxing between beats. Half the blood goes to the lungs for oxygen. The other half has already been there and is now pumped out into the rest of the body. The double thump you hear is the sound of valves opening and closing at the top and bottom of the heart to allow all this to happen.

The heart beats and the blood moves on. We can't live without it. There was a chance that Martin's healthy young heart might work for Marc in a way that his own defeated, swollen heart no longer could.

The retrieval team told the surgeon waiting up at the Freeman Hospital in Newcastle that all was well and he could start preparing his patient. They used a clamp to stop the flow of blood into the heart and injected a chilling solution of potassium to slow down the beat then make it stop, in much the same way as had been done for the first ever transplant back in

1967. Martin was already dead, legally speaking, but now his life also came to an end in the traditional sense, as his heart beat for the last time. The surgeons were focused on the next step, though. Their aim was to bring this one part of him back. They were going to remove and transport the heart then revive it inside the body of a complete stranger, in the hope of giving that person many more years – if they could just get it to Marc in time.

The clock was ticking from the moment the heart was clamped. When the beating stopped, the four tubes carrying blood to and from the body were cut and the heart was disconnected, lifted out of the chest cavity and carried across the room carefully by a nurse in gloves and a mask, to be packed in salt water in a sterile bag inside another sterile bag inside a third sterile bag and packed with ice in a protective white plastic box with a carrier handle, marked in blue with the words 'Human Tissue'.

They had four hours to get the heart from Nottingham to Newcastle and into Marc before it began to deteriorate. After that it would quickly become useless.

The body of Martin Burton was sewn up after the operation and brought back to the intensive care unit. A nurse bent over him there, cleaning the iodine from his bruised skin, washing his hair and tending for him as if he was still alive, before he went off to the Chapel of Rest. Harish Vyas finished his rounds, checking up on all the children in his care, before he could allow himself to leave at three in the morning. He felt the loss of Martin and knew what was coming.

'Usually I become silent when we lose a child. I go home and remain silent for a while, I don't talk to anyone, not even to my own kids. That is probably me gradually grieving in my own way. I don't communicate with anyone for a day or two and then I come out of it and back to my normal self.'

Long after Martin Burton had gone to theatre to have his heart removed and prepared for the journey to Newcastle, the consultant drove home exhausted. He pulled over and stopped his car at the top of the hill overlooking his village, with the deep, peaceful darkness of the countryside stretching out ahead of him down below. He got out, stretched his back and took a deep breath, through his nose, filling his lungs with the first fresh air after the long days and nights inside the hospital.

The next day he stayed at home alone, as was his custom after losing a patient. He was very quiet, even when the children came home. They found him kneading dough and rolling it out for home-made pizzas, with fresh tomato and mozzarella ready, and they all knew what that meant. 'In my silent phase, I make pizzas. I feed my family. It is a way of finishing the day by at least doing something for my children, overcoming the grief by showing there is still life. They have got to know after a while that if I make pizzas and I am quiet, something dastardly has happened at work.'

The ritual was so familiar that Harish Vyas sometimes had to take steps to avoid making his children become alarmed at the sight of a home-made thin-crust pepperoni. 'Occasionally I make pizzas without any dastardly things happening. I have to do that, so they don't get scared every time they see me rolling out the dough.'

The blood supply to Martin's heart was cut off with the clamp at two-thirty in the morning on Friday 29 August, but it took time to remove and prepare the heart, which did not leave the hospital until just after three-thirty. Now there were only three hours left to reach Marc. That wasn't quite enough. The journey from Nottingham to Newcastle by road would take three hours even with the blue lights flashing and no traffic all the way up the A1. They were cutting it too fine.

Lynne Holt had already anticipated this and been in touch with a private transport company to book a plane – so the driver of the car carrying the heart turned south first, against instinct, and sped through the early hours of the morning to East Midlands Airport, a dozen miles away. There he took the back road, fast-tracked by airport security to the south apron, where a light aircraft was waiting with a pair of turbo-driven propellers already turning.

Once the box had been lifted from the car to the back of the plane and secured with just the two members of the aircraft crew for company, the pilot opened the throttle and began to taxi for take-off. The wind was picking up that night as fiercely cold air came in from the Arctic to blow the summer away, so it took longer than expected to fly up the spine of the country, with the shadowed contours of the Yorkshire Moors down on the left and the North York Moors on the right. This was a short flight, but nothing was guaranteed. Planes do crash. A whole transplant team died a few years ago when an air ambulance for a heart patient came down and exploded in Nevada. A Cessna carrying a liver from Belfast to Birmingham crash-landed in autumn fog more recently and caught fire with the pilot inside. The fireman who pulled him out also rescued the white transplant box, so the operation could go ahead and another life was saved. 'I've gone over it and over it and over it, waking up at night and thinking about it,' he said later. 'Luckily for us, everything went well.'

The surgeons in Newcastle would not begin to remove Marc's heart until they knew the plane carrying the new one had touched down and was safely on the ground.

'The weather does keep the adrenaline going,' says Lynne, the lead transplant co-ordinator, who was walking back and forth between the operating theatre and her office in scrubs, taking calls and letting the surgeon know what was going on. Timing was everything. The switch of hearts had to be done as quickly as possible to avoid a disaster. 'The surgeon was waiting for that heart to come through the door.'

The box was carried down the steps from the plane and put into an ambulance waiting on the tarmac at Newcastle International Airport, a mile from the terminal, where commuters in suits were already waiting for the Friday red-eye shuttle to London and tourists in shorts and straw hats were arriving dazed from sunnier places.

The time was a quarter to six in the morning. There were now only forty-five minutes left to get the heart into Marc. The hospital was seven miles away by road. That would take half an hour in normal traffic, twenty minutes with a police escort. Marc's mother and father had been awake there all night. So had Lynne. 'There was a lot of stress, all totally understandable. Families in a situation like that haven't slept for days, they're not eating, they're not drinking, so just trying to get some toast and tea into them is as much as we can hope for. I try and explain that we need them to be fit for when their son wakes up after the operation, but they never think of themselves, all they think of is him.'

There was no way Linda was going to sleep while her son was in surgery. 'I had been pacing the corridors all night, I was actually outside the theatre just standing there, staring at the doors for a while. I couldn't see anything, but there was this urge to be near him.'

She asked if she could go in to watch the operation. The staff said no, in the nicest possible way, so Linda kept pacing and ran into Norrie, who was doing the same thing. They went outside together for a smoke and were standing by the front entrance to the hospital in the dawn light when familiar flickers of blue suddenly appeared on the glass of the windows and shelters around them, reflecting the lights of the police car that was pulling up, almost silently, with an ambulance behind.

'There's another poor soul,' said Norrie, wearily. Linda heard the wheeze of the hospital's automatic doors behind her and a transplant nurse came out in her surgical gown, straight from theatre: 'Linda, here comes Marc's new heart.'

Marc's mother's legs gave way suddenly and she found herself on the pavement, on her knees, being helped up, unable to quite comprehend what she was looking at. 'It was in a box like you would take on a picnic with your sandwiches and cold cans in.'

Then it was gone.

Five past six. They had just twenty-five minutes to get the heart to theatre and connect it up, which was very tight timing indeed. Lynne Holt took the heart from the driver and was tempted to run, but she walked very briskly instead so as not to drop the box and ruin everything at the last moment. 'I put the box onto a trolley and just pulled it through the hospital on wheels, that was the easy part.'

The surgeon and his team had also been up all night, preparing for an operation that was going to take all day. Even if their hands were sure and swift, even if the organ was undamaged by the journey, even if the body did not reject the heart, Marc might still not be strong enough to survive. After all this effort by so many people, he might yet die on the operating table.

Linda did not know what was going on behind the closed doors and there was nothing she could do about it. All her nervous energy had to go somewhere, so she fretted about the donor and his family. All she knew was they were from the Midlands. 'I was think-ing about this wee boy of sixteen and his mum and dad have just lost him and they've let his heart go to somebody they don't even know. How can they be doing this? They don't even know who we are, what kind of people we are. What better gift can you give people than life? I just felt so humble. I was grieving for them as well, but worrying for Marc. We weren't out of the woods.'

FOURTEEN

MARC

The surgeon stood to the right of Marc's body with his gloved hands in the air, ready to begin. This would be a tricky operation, but Leslie Hamilton was used to that. The handsome fifty-something Northern Irishman with a super-calm manner and soothing voice was one of the best heart surgeons in the country, and perhaps the very best at carrying out transplants for children. Heart surgeons are the rock stars of medicine, but he has a way of laughing that off. 'We're plumbers. We just connect the pipes.' Plumbers can turn the water off before they start to work, though. The water isn't blood. The house isn't a living human being who will die if they get it wrong.

Mr Hamilton had done a full day's work at the Freeman on Thursday before popping home for tea and coming back about midnight. Marc had gone into theatre at that time to be examined and prepared as the surgical team got everything ready, then waited for the word from Nottingham that the heart was coming. Now it was definitely on its way. The surgeon wore loose-fitting green surgical scrubs and cap, a face mask and heavy, black-rimmed glasses with curious magnifying lenses that appeared to have been cut off a pair of binoculars. A headlight strapped to his fore-head would help him see the way into the heart. There were half a dozen others in the room, including a perfusionist to check the blood supply going through the heart-lung machine that would keep Marc McCay alive while his own heart was removed and another stitched in.

Mr Hamilton looked around at his team.

'Shall we make a start?'

He was used to pressure. There are few sharper ways to learn how to stay calm than working in casualty in Belfast at the height of the Troubles as Leslie Hamilton did. Bombs, guns, beatings and kneecappings, the victims all came to the hospital on the Falls Road where he helped out as a medical student in his youth. Loyalists, Republicans, gunmen or innocent bystanders, they all ended up at the same hospital. There, among the blood and guts, he realised that the attitude of the best medics was always the same: 'Faced with a difficult situation, you analyse it and deal with it first. Reflect on it later.'

The first time he opened a human body up to fix a problem inside the chest, he knew this was his thing. '"Wow," I thought. "This is what I want to do." The excitement of it all, the drama of the patient deteriorating rapidly, you've got to make decisions fast and if you do the right thing it works.'

Mr Hamilton went on to work in Leeds and at Great Ormond Street Hospital, building his reputation and specialising in children in the early days of heart surgery in Britain. 'Lots of patients died at the beginning. We didn't have the sophisticated blood tests and clotting products we have now and they had to be really sick, with no other alternatives, before they were referred to us. I learned from a generation of senior surgeons who had to be slightly mad to keep going.'

The pressure then was immense. Any child might die under the knife and any slip of the hand might kill them. 'It's a very fine line you walk between confidence in yourself and arrogance, and some people tip over onto the arrogant side. It's self-protection. Once you start doubting yourself it is time to stop. A couple of deaths can destroy you, psychologically.'

Mr Hamilton had been at the Freeman for a dozen years by the time he stood over the sedated body of Marc McCay. His own son was twenty-two years old and his daughters were twenty, eighteen and fifteen. He was just into his fifties, and well aware that he had been an absent father. 'When he was young, my son said, "Can't somebody else's daddy look after the sick babies for a while?"' But there were very few surgeons doing what he did and he felt a strong emotional connection to his patients. 'When you see a young person coming in for transplant who has been cut down in their prime as Marc was, that is really difficult.'

Even if Marc McCay survived the operation and his body did not reject the heart immediately, there was a strong chance he would die within a year. Then again he would die much sooner if they did nothing. This boy was as close to death as anyone could be, but Leslie Hamilton might have it in his fingers, his brain and his power to save his life. 'Why do children's heart surgery? Because the rewards of seeing a child get back to normal and live a full life again ... it doesn't get any better than that.'

He had to cut his way into Marc's chest to get to the heart. That meant scoring a line down the centre of the breastbone with an electrical saw then sawing right through, being careful to stay in the middle. 'If you cut through the ribs by mistake it would be messy trying to put the bits of that jigsaw back together again afterwards.' Smoke rose from the lining of the bone as he burnt it to stop the bleeding. Then Mr Hamilton used a hand-cranked metal spreader, like a clamp in reverse, to pull the two halves of the breastbone apart and keep them in place with its claws. The whole thing was as brutal as butchery, but more precise.

The heart is enclosed in a white, oily, shiny but leathery sack called a pericardium, so he cut that open – but the surgeon did not start to remove Marc's swollen heart from the body until he knew that the air ambulance had touched down and the new heart was on its way to the hospital by road, a journey from the airport of about twenty minutes. 'We didn't want to take any chances about that.'

The four natural tubes that lead into and out of the heart were now clamped to stop the flow of blood and so a machine was officially doing the job of the heart completely, as it actually had been for Marc since he first got to the hospital. The old organ was slowly cut away and lifted out. 'Marc was so sick, his heart was so much bigger than would have been the normal heart in a sixteen-year-old. Sometimes we can retrieve the valves and use them in heart surgery for other patients, but this was just one big flabby bag of very thinned-out muscle.'

Lynne Holt rushed into the operating theatre, wheeling the picnic box with the new heart behind her, and could see the old one was a mess. 'It was lying there in a bowl, just so damaged. Quite often, hearts still beat for five or ten minutes after they have been removed from the body, but that did not happen this time. Marc's old heart did not beat. It didn't really look like a heart at all.'

Martin's heart was also lifeless at that moment, as it was lifted off the ice in the box and put in a silver metal bowl. The first of the three clear plastic bags was cut open and the scalpel thrown away, because it was no longer sterile. Then the next bag was opened, and the next, until Mr Hamilton could see the heart was healthy and there was a good chance this was going to work if he did his job right. 'We were ready to start sewing in the new heart as soon as it came out of the box.'

The clunky magnifying lenses made his glasses heavy, but he was used to that. He needed them to see the fine thread, like fishing line, with which he would sew the plugs of the new heart to the pipes of Marc's body. The first connection to be made was on the back of the organ as it was going to sit in the body, so the assistant held the heart over Marc's chest, tilted on its side in his hand. 'You have to make sure you don't get anything twisted,' says the surgeon, who made the first stitches then slid the heart down into place in the chest cavity, after a careful check. 'You want to make sure your stitches are in the right place so they don't bleed afterwards where you can't get to them without taking out the whole heart again.'

The front of the heart was next, including the aorta – the main artery that takes blood away to the rest of the body. 'We hadn't finished the transplant but we did take the clamp off and allow Marc's blood to flow backwards into the new heart at that point, because what happens next speeds the whole operation up and is truly extraordinary, even for me. I never get tired of seeing it.'

The new heart was still cold, yellow and lifeless, still full of the potassium solution that had been used to stop it back in Nottingham, a little over four hours earlier. This fluid is used to enact the death penalty and stop the hearts of murderers in America, but what was about to happen here was a reverse execution. A heart coming back from death to life.

Blood flowed into the new heart, flushing out the potassium and slowly warming up the organ. The colour began to change in response, from white and blue to pink and red. Then suddenly, without any help, there was a twitch in the meaty muscle. A tiny convulsion. Then another. A wait and then another, growing in strength and regularity until the new heart was suddenly beating away fully in the open chest. Ba-boom again. Ba-boom.

This looked miraculous, even to an experienced surgeon who knew what was happening and why. 'It's a natural phenomenon. The heart has a natural pacemaker within itself, a small area of tissue that sends an electrical impulse to the rest of the heart and makes it beat.'

The electricity is created in the first place by a chemical reaction in the blood, but that's the science. Feelings are something else. Leslie Hamilton has a cool command of his subject, but he does become emotional when he talks about the wonder of a transplant. 'When you start training in surgery and you take a heart out for the first time, you see this big space in the middle of the body where the heart used to be and you think, "This is crazy." Then you put in the new heart and it fills the space but it is this little, collapsed bag sitting there, flaccid and empty. You take the clamp off and see the blood go in and it changes colour. You get the first couple of beats that start, then it becomes a better rhythm and suddenly it just starts to beat normally. It's an amazing thing.'

His voice cracks as he remembers how that happened to Martin's heart as it lay in Marc. 'It was cold, it was motionless and doing absolutely nothing and then it was full of blood and beating … that is one of the most amazing sights in surgery.'

* * *

Elation had to wait. There was a complication. Marc's old heart had swollen so much that the pipes into his body had been pushed back and the new heart was too small to fit. The surgeon had to fill in the gaps with patches made from the lining of a cow's heart. Now was the time to find out if this was all going to work, by weaning Marc off the machine that had been keeping him alive between hearts. Slowly, the perfusionist sitting behind Mr Hamilton reduced the pace at which it was pumping blood, until Marc's new heart was doing all the work. 'That's the moment of truth. Sometimes the heart just blows up like a balloon and you know you've got problems.'

The team waited. Twenty anxious minutes.

'Even when the perfusionist has switched the heart-lung machine off, we wait for a while with the tubes still in place, just in case. When we are happy, we take out the tubes and wait for another while. If that's okay, we close up his chest and take him back to intensive care.'

The surgeon had to decide whether to let his colleagues close up the body so he could go down to the ward to see the family. 'You don't want to go too early. You don't want to get your fingers burned. The last thing you want to do is go and give them false reassurance.' He did once tell a couple that their newborn had died, when behind him in the operating theatre his team was watching the little baby come back to life. 'In Marc's case, the heart worked well and everything seemed fine.'

Marc left the operating theatre just before noon on the Friday, twelve hours after going in. He would still be on a ventilator for his lungs for at least the next twelve hours and in a coma for quite a while yet before he was allowed to surface, and that would be full of risks too. Some patients still die in the first few days after a heart transplant, although not as many are lost as there used to be. It's still a huge, traumatic operation that tests the will to survive both mentally and physically. One in five heart transplant patients die in the first year. Half die within a decade, says Leslie Hamilton, although younger people are slightly more likely to survive: half of them will go on for at least fourteen years.

'We don't know which ones will survive and which will die. One of the difficulties is that death is seen as a failure of medical treatment, but there is a time when it is natural to die. With Marc, it was about watching and waiting for nature to take its course, allowing the healing process to kick into action and supporting his body over the next few days. His kidneys had been hurt by the fact that his heart was so sick. Marc was going to take a very long time to recover fully. If he ever did.'

FIFTEEN

MARTIN

Sue's parents, Len and Joan, drove her and Nigel home to Grantham, to the neat detached house with the flowers in boxes outside and the cat sniffing around wondering where everybody was and Martin's shoes in the hallway and his cuddly toys all still lined up on the bottom bunk in his room. The scent of him was still in there, all as it was before his death, and Nigel and Sue walked past it all as if in a trance and got into bed together and slept.

They were completely exhausted, way beyond shattered, having been up for days and lived through the most traumatic times of both their lives, facing the worst heartbreak a parent can endure and finally they slept. They slept like they had never slept before and would never sleep again. But Martin woke them up early. It wasn't really him, of course, but it was coming from his bedroom. The sound of his alarm going off at five past eight on the Friday morning. The sound that wouldn't stop. Nigel couldn't work out where it was coming from or what the hell was happening but then he realised through his fog that the sound was an echo of Martin. He had set his alarm when he went to bed that night because he was heading for college to enrol the next day and it must have gone off every day while they were in hospital because here it was, going off again and again. And again.

'I rushed through to the bedroom and killed the alarm but the damage had been done. Then it all came back to me, vividly. Our son had died. He was dead. He wasn't there. It wasn't a terrible dream that we could snap out of, it was real. Horrible.'

He felt like smashing the alarm clock. 'I wasn't angry at the actual clock but it was the focus for the situation we were in and there was this intense anger at the taking of the life of a healthy sixteen-year-old who had everything ahead of him and I was just left with this emotionless grief. It took a lot of control to just turn off that clock and put it back down on the window ledge.'

They did not know this at the time, but the alarm went off around the time Martin's heart was beginning to beat inside Marc, hundreds of miles away.

Sue woke up bewildered and in real physical pain. 'At first, you honestly wonder how you are going to

119

live with a grief that is so intense. We were only in our forties; I imagined I would always feel how I felt that first morning, I didn't think it would ever change and I just didn't know how I was going to deal with it.'

Heartbreak is real. It hurts like the heart is actually breaking. Like a burning, like a chilling, like a scream under the ribcage. The aching. The shock. The numbness. The nausea. The tiredness. All at once. Like electricity in the veins. Like the weeping that will not come, because tears are not enough. Sue was raging at the world for being so cruel but she kept it all locked inside her, like a bomb going off in her chest. She couldn't eat, her stomach was churning and anyway nothing tasted of anything anymore. She couldn't sleep, her mind was continuously replaying the night of Martin's collapse and it just would not stop. Someone would be talking to her and she would not be listening, she'd be reliving those moments, without wanting to. Over and over again. It was exhausting. She couldn't concentrate on anything, couldn't settle.

Nigel was in his own world too. They were avoiding each other, treading on eggshells as they paced around their house that suddenly felt so empty. These were sensible, resourceful people, but death unravels us all. 'We just crashed. You just don't function after a thing like that. You don't want to eat, you don't want to cook, you don't want to shop. You don't want to get up, get washed, get dressed. You just want to sit there. You can't think for yourself. You're in shock.'

They did try to get on with things that needed doing over that weekend, but it was impossible. 'There's this emotion that hits you again and you just stop in your tracks, sit down and go back into tears at the realisation that your son has gone, you won't see him again.'

Sue was usually so busy, but now she just stopped too. 'I remember spending hours just staring out of the window at nothing. A lot of deep sighing is common in that very early stage of grief. We tried to be good parents, we'd brought our children up well. I didn't understand why we were being put through this.'

Standing in the kitchen, she noticed blood on the knuckles of her eldest son's hands and snapped at him. 'What have you been doing?' Christopher was reluctant to say. Nothing, he said, but it wasn't true. 'He'd been outside thumping the wall,' remembers Sue, who was troubled. This was really not like him at all. 'Chris was – and still is – the most laid-back, peaceful-natured boy. I don't think he ever thumped anybody in his life but both his hands were bleeding, which was awful.'

She knew what was going on and it cut through the numbness to make her feel again, hurting for her big boy. 'He was at the worst possible age to lose his brother, having just turned twenty. If he had been younger, he would have shown his emotions another way: children can't help it, they cry. If he had been older, he would have been able to talk about it and thrash it through that way. Young males of that age can't show their emotions, they don't get upset and cry, they get frustrated and angry. I just wanted to give him a hug and let him cry but he wouldn't. You can't change people and that was his nature then, awful for him though it all was.'

Nigel understood why Christopher was so angry. 'He always protected Martin. He always tried to look after him and he defended Martin sometimes on things that weren't defendable, but that was his instinct. So he was in this position where something terrible had happened to his little brother and there was nothing he could do about it and that frustrated him so much.'

As a father, Nigel also felt guilty that he wasn't able to give Christopher what he needed at that moment. 'The bottom had just fallen out of my world. You feel sorry because you have another son but at that moment in time your sole focus is on the child you've just lost and what's happening to him and what could've happened – what he could have done in life – and your loss, the things you're going to miss out on now you've lost him. You think, "How do we put this back together and how do we have a life?" How does a life resume after such an all-consuming loss? Losing a child is a terrible thing to have to happen to any parent, it grips you really hard and you think, "How do I climb out of this hole?"

'Initially, you don't think you will. It takes weeks and months before the light starts to come and you see where you're going to go and how you'll proceed. That's when friends really do help. It's hard to do even the simple things like cook, so our friends brought food round – shepherd's pie, lasagne – just to keep us going. They would sit there and hold your hand and let you weep and cry and they would just be there for you. That's what you need at that time.'

Christopher had Ashley and she was a huge help, says Sue. 'She was only eighteen at the time so she had a lot to contend with, but Ashley stuck to Chris like glue and went through everything with him, every step of the way. I will always be grateful for the way she was over those days, and her family as well. They were amazing to him.'

So the Burtons had people around who could help that weekend after Martin's death and that was good, because they were going to need them. There were very challenging days to come.

SIXTEEN

MARC

He's in a fish tank, thought Leasa. She was looking through the thick glass of the window into the isolation unit on the high dependency ward, because the nurses wouldn't let her in to see her brother. Only Mum and Dad could go in through the double-door airlock and they had to wear plastic gowns. If they had any sniffles, they had to stay out in case he got an infection. She stood there all morning feeling self-conscious, staring into the room with little awareness of the bustle of activity around her, although when trolleys came past her backside she had to squeeze in with her nose to the glass. Everything was clinical and white in there, but the weak light from the strips in the ceiling and an outside window on the far side of the bed gave it all a strange, sickly, greeny-blue colour, like the water in an aquarium.

Marc was connected to a heart monitor, and there were tubes into his neck, his arm, his groin and in his nose. A bigger one down his throat was helping him to breathe. Mum was in there – she had pulled up the armchair to the end of his bed and was holding his feet. She'd lost a couple of stone since Marc got sick, Leasa could see that. Mum wasn't sleeping and had refused to take any more sleeping tablets since that second morning, when Ryan had to wake her up. 'I wanted to sleep, honest I did, because if I could sleep then none of this would be happening,' remembers Linda. 'I could block it all out. But I didn't want to go to sleep, at the same time, because I wanted to be there for Marc. I didn't want to miss a single thing.'

She had to be careful where she moved in order to not jog anything or pull it out by accident so her back was burning as she sat by his bed for hours, stroking his forehead, holding his hand and talking to him about his sixteenth birthday that was coming up soon. Without even thinking about it, she was focusing on the future, willing him to get there. 'Marc, what do you want for your birthday, darling? It's your birthday next week, you can have anything you want. Do you want a surprise? I know you love surprises.' She would break down in tears for a while, before starting up again. 'Marc, you're needing a haircut.'

The nurses were quiet behind her, she could tell something was wrong.

'Have you seen him move, Linda? There, on his right side?'

She hadn't, come to think of it. But she couldn't be sure.

'Okay. We'll do some tests. He's under sedation, but still …'

His left foot twitched under Linda's hand, but not the right. The test results came back and revealed that Marc had suffered a stroke which had partially paralysed his right side. Linda became hysterical, rushing out of the room to find her daughter, who tried to calm her down. 'I don't know what I would have done without Leasa,' she says now. 'When I settled a bit I was thinking, "I don't care if he's had a stroke and his right side doesn't work, because he's still here and he's still my Marc. I've still got him, after everything that has happened. I'll cope. I have to."'

SEVENTEEN

MARTIN

So now Sue and Nigel had to register Martin's death, to make it official. The stroke of a pen, a mark on a page, the facts of the matter and a couple of signatures. The boy whose birth had been recorded in Grantham in April 1987 was now to become another entry on a different register, far too soon. That meant Sue and Nigel driving back to Nottingham only a few days after they had left him there, which was tough. By now, though, the pair of them were so mummified by layer upon layer of grief, sadness and anger and who knows what other emotions that they had almost ceased to feel anything. Almost. Until they walked into the register office on the Monday. 'There was this young lady sitting behind a desk and all around her on the walls were pictures that had been done by her kids. She did not appreciate what was going on. In front of her was a couple who had just lost a child and these pictures were reminding us of our loss,' says Sue, who was thrown by what she saw. 'She should have taken us into a neutral office. I thought that was the most uncaring, thoughtless act.'

Martin's body was taken to the Chapel of Rest at the offices of Robert Holland, a friend of the family who had been an independent funeral director in the town for more than two decades. His own son knew Martin and she remembers that what Mr Holland said was kind. 'Come any time of day, or in the night if you need to. Just give us a call and a couple of minutes to get prepared for you, but do come.'

She did not want to go to see Martin in his coffin at all, but Nigel knew it was necessary. 'The last time I had seen my son he was warm, he was pink, he was breathing. I had to go and see him again to put in my mind, finally, that he was dead. It's not pleasant to have to view your child like that but I felt I had to finalise the thing.'

Sue was persuaded to go with Nigel by a friend who happened to be a nurse. 'I didn't think I would cope, but she pointed out that if I didn't go to see Martin then my lasting memories would be of him wired up to life support. She encouraged me to go and see him looking like himself in his own clothes without all the tubes and things.'

Sue was afraid of the state he would be in after the organ retrieval, but Robert Holland insisted it would be fine, he would make sure that she did not see anything she could not cope with. 'On those grounds, I agreed to go.'

They had sorted out a pair of jeans and a football shirt for Martin to wear in his coffin. 'We sent a West Ham cap so that any head injuries could be covered up and the funeral director told us that because he had donated his corneas, each of his eyes would be closed with just a small stitch.'

You could hardly see those stitches, says Sue. 'If anybody else had looked in and seen him, they would not have noticed immediately that there was anything different about him. He looked very pale, very cold, but at least he was in his own clothes rather than a hospital gown. In that sense, he looked like Martin.'

They were not alone at the Chapel of Rest. Her mother and father, Len and Joan, came too and Joan almost collapsed when they entered the room, remembers Sue. 'We were trying to hold her up.'

Christopher was there and this time he did cry, at the sight of his baby brother looking so strange. Sue and Ashley hugged him together.

Afterwards, when they were back at home, Sue told Nigel that she had been thinking. It was good for them to do that together as a family, but would he mind if they went back? 'I felt I had to go for a second time later, just with my husband. Without anyone else. We didn't even tell anyone we were going.'

So the next day they were able to stand quietly alone together in the Chapel of Rest in the presence of their son, too numb to know what they were thinking or feeling. It was only later that Sue would reflect on how this moment helped her understand, at last, deep inside herself, that these were his remains and the Martin she knew and loved so much was no longer there.

'I needed my time. I didn't want to have to worry about my mother, I didn't want to have to worry about Christopher, I had to go for me. I had to stand there, look at Martin and establish in my own mind that this was for real.'

A letter from the transplant nurse at the hospital arrived before Martin had even been buried, letting them know what had happened to the parts of his body that had been taken away. 'Firstly, may I pass on my sincere condolences to you all at this time. I would like to take this opportunity to thank you for allowing Martin to become an organ donor, it was an incredibly brave decision of yours.'

His heart, lungs, liver and both kidneys had been used. The pancreas was inflamed and disposed of, but that was not unusual. They knew this meant it had been incinerated. There were no children with the right blood type who needed a kidney, so patients had been chosen from the adult waiting list. 'Martin's left kidney was transplanted into a sixty-one-year-old man. He has a daughter and a grand-daughter aged eighteen years. The co-ordinator involved with his care has informed me that he is extremely grateful for the opportunity of a more normal life that you have given to him, and his new kidney is working well.'

The right kidney had gone to a fifty-five-year-old lady, but there was no more information about that yet. Nor did the transplant nurse know anything about the man who had received his lungs. The liver had helped a thirty-four-year-old man suffering with an extremely rare liver condition, who was now recovering well. He was married with two children. Martin's eyes were being stored for future use.

Then there was the heart.

'Martin was able to donate his heart to a fifteen-year-old boy, who had suffered from a condition known as cardiomyopathy and was desperately ill. He has woken up since his operation, obviously he has a long recovery ahead.'

That was all the letter said about his condition, which the doctors had also called myocarditis, but the letter finished with a personal note from the nurse who had written it.

I cannot imagine the suffering you are going through at this time and I only hope this information will be of some small comfort to you in the future. Martin has allowed five persons the opportunity of life-saving or life-enhancing transplants, I am sure you must be very proud of him. It was a privilege to spend time with Martin and to meet you. I hope you will feel able to contact me if there is anything I can help you with. You are very special people, it would be nice to help you as you have selflessly helped others.

That was comfort to Sue, but quite honestly, she could barely take it all in. The funeral was coming. Then she would really have to let him go.

EIGHTEEN

MARC

Marc walked beside his father, down by the river. The sunlight slipped between the leaves of the trees, falling down on them like golden rain as they talked about this and that. The football and the weather, everything and nothing, Norrie and Marc just shooting the breeze as father and son, but there was another man beside them. Marc's grandfather, a proud, straight-backed man in a crisp white shirt and dark blazer from the bowls club, walking with a measured step, head down as if pacing out the distance to the jack.

'Y'all right, son?' he said to Marc, nodding before the answer. Marc's grandfather was not a man to suffer fools gladly, he was self-contained and severe. He knew his opinions and backed his own judgement, and he valued the respect of his peers as the foreman at an engineering company. They called him Mr McCay, never by his first name, but Marc knew him as Grampa, the man of the house, the head of the family, who was walking with them by the river.

'See this right, there's someone I want you to meet,' said Norrie, slowing down and stopping, and there standing under a tree, leaning against the trunk, in a black three-piece suit with a high collar and tie from the old days was a pear-shaped man, pale and a little wheezy, but with a certain dignity. 'This is your great-grampa.'

Marc took the hand that was offered to him and wondered how his great-grampa and grampa could be the same age, and he was surprised when the man spoke. 'What about ye?' His accent was a little Irish, warm and friendly but precise in his diction. 'Glad to see ye. I've heard your troubles, son. I hear ye can play.'

Marc said, 'Yes, up front.' His great-grandfather smiled. 'Ah. Inside-forward? Aye. Good. Strength, agility, pace. Courage, too. You will be needing that. There's a big match ahead, a big match ahead. You're a Hun, then?' Marc laughed, recognising an old nickname for the followers of Rangers. 'I am John McCay, by the way.'

Marc was startled by the way he pronounced his name, to rhyme with eye. He knew nothing at all about the Edwardian gentleman he was talking to, but that was no surprise. They had never met before, because John McCay had been dead for twenty-two years. Marc was lying in a hospital bed in Newcastle in a coma, yet still here they were, speaking together. It seemed so real, but this was actually a dream he had while unconscious, probably in the high dependency unit after his operation. Marc was kept deep in the coma and on the ventilator for a day after surgery to allow his body to recover, and in case anything went wrong and they needed to put him back under fast. Then the drugs were reduced gradually over the next few days to allow him to surface slowly. When he did eventually come round, Marc would remember the dream, vividly.

'I wish you well then. Pleasure to meet you, son,' said the old man. 'I'll be waiting for ye, but I'm gonnae put ye back with your Mum and your Dad now …'

And with that, Marc woke up.

NINETEEN

MARTIN

What song should Martin have at his funeral? His parents asked his friends, who picked something he would have loved. Not a soppy song like 'Wind Beneath My Wings' or one of the oldies like Frank Sinatra singing 'My Way' but a happy, catchy cover of 'The Tide is High' by Atomic Kitten, a glossy pop trio who were in the charts. 'He was very much into Atomic Kitten, which was more to do with the attractive young ladies than with the music,' says Nigel fondly. 'That was a very popular song at the time. Music for Martin was quite easy.'

The funeral was held on a Friday afternoon in early September 2003, just eight days after Martin's death. They had to make their choices quickly, says Sue, but that was a mercy. 'You are still in your bubble of shock, that's what protects you through all the preparations. How on earth can you sit and discuss with somebody what you want in the service when it has been a sudden death and it's your own child? But you do have to choose music and what he is going to wear and it was good to get it done.' They went for a simple service with words and songs familiar to them: 'The Lord of the Dance', as heard in many a school assembly, the traditional version of The Lord's Prayer and the hymn 'Lord of All Hopefulness', with its plea for God to be 'there at our sleeping' and grant peace. 'If the funeral had been six weeks later I think we would have gone to pieces over the decisions, because by then you just don't want to go there. Grief has really set in.'

His friends turned up in force. There were a couple of hundred teenagers at the funeral, standing around outside the Grantham crematorium before the service, in clusters in the chilly air, the girls dabbing at their eyes, the boys trying to look as if they had not also been crying. Most were in the uniform of Sir William Robertson Academy, a navy blue blazer, white shirt and black trousers or a black skirt. 'That was humbling, to see how many of Martin's peers had come to pay their final respects to our son', remembers Sue. 'They were everywhere, it really hit home. He was such a well-liked person. They still remember his birthday and his death day, the mates he had then.

They take flowers up to the Garden of Remembrance. They're very good.'

The room was simple but elegant, with wooden chairs, bare walls, high windows and a slatted wooden ceiling. The funeral attendants squeezed in as many mourners as they safely could. It was a difficult morning, even for them. Their job was to help things go smoothly and not be noticed, but by terrible coincidence that day they were serving at the cremation of two young men of similar ages, one after another. Some of the teenagers were there for both services, says Sue. 'We know the other family very well now, the son died while they were on holiday.'

Martin's coffin rested on a plinth where the altar would have been in a church. The heavy curtain on either side of the recess made it feel more like a stage. Nigel was in a daze until right at the end of the service. 'You don't see the coffin go off, they just close the curtains around it and that is horrible, it is the final moment.'

'It's one of those final moments,' says Sue quietly. 'There seem to be so many.'

There's always an awkward silence at the end of a funeral service when nobody really knows what to do. Should we stand up yet? Is it okay to talk? So people sit there and pull out mints to suck, or bow their heads for a moment more of silent prayer or just stare at the Order of Service, waiting for release. This time it came with the crash of tinny drums and a swirl of cheap synthesiser, as the song Christopher had chosen for his brother began to play in the speakers. A tune everyone knew instantly, but some couldn't quite believe they were hearing. First the unexpected sound of a cheering crowd then a cheesy reggae backing track and a rough choir, singing like they were on the terraces. 'I'm forever blowing bubbles, pretty bubbles in the air …'

The big brother who was a Forest fan had chosen the West Ham theme song for his sibling, his little mate. They'd joked and sparred about football many times, and played in the park in their clashing team shirts, half tackling and half wrestling but always laughing and teasing. Now Chris had brought all that happy rivalry into the funeral room, in such a daft, unexpected way that it made people smile, look around, breathe out, relax.

'It was such a tinny, Seventies sort of music and it was on repeat while everyone was filing out of the chapel so it played half a dozen times and seemed to get tinnier every time. The whole thing lifted the mood, which I felt was very important for the young people there. I could hear one or two of them tittering,' says Sue. They glanced across at her, feeling guilty for wanting to laugh, but she did her best to smile back. It was okay, she would have said if she had been capable of any kind of speech at that moment. Martin would have cracked some silly joke about it all, to break the tension. That was the whole point, says Nigel. 'It was a way to represent Martin and to give his friends something to laugh about. Martin would have liked that.'

TWENTY

MARC

Marc had passed out in a battered old hospital in Glasgow, but now he began to wake up in some alien place, a futuristic room full of technology that looked like it belonged in a spaceship. He was hurting all over, but he was floating too and he couldn't understand what was happening. Then he was sleeping again. He was in a shop, with a big plate glass window. A bed shop, maybe. No, Blackpool with his football team and this was a hotel, he was on his back in the hotel room, looking over at the window. That was his sister, Leasa, outside looking in. Waving at him. She was waving at him, with his brothers, Darren and Ryan. Where was his mum? He tried to call out, but there was something on his face. He was bound tight like a mummy or it felt that way, his arms tied tight to his side or maybe they were heavy, just heavy. Aye, they were heavy like lead and his feet too. Heavy.

The light in the shop was bright, but there was a shadow, a figure, a sinister figure moving about, coming closer. A woman with a uniform on, blue like the Rangers strip, but she wasn't a friend, she had a look in her eye like a killer. She was saying something and her accent was English, why was she English? She was coming for him with a needle, a huge needle, as big as a skewer. It was going into his arm, into his skin, he could see the puncture mark and the liquid going in. She was poisoning him, the woman was killing him and Leasa was waving but Marc was dying here, he was dying, he was dying away and where was his mum?

'Mum!' No sound came out. 'Mum!'

'It took a long while to get through to him,' says Linda, who was there with his father Norrie when Marc came round properly a few days after the operation, just as his great grampa had promised in the dream he would eventually remember as if it was real. For the moment, he was drifting in and out of consciousness. 'I thought Marc was awake and I was trying to explain everything to him, but I would say something and he would go back to sleep. It took days for me to realise he didn't know what I was talking about.'

The nurse rolled him towards her when she was changing the bed and Linda got close up to her son's face and kissed him and told him about what had happened. He had passed out in hospital in Scotland but that was nearly a fortnight ago and now he was in Newcastle and they were all looking after him. 'Sweetheart, you've had a heart transplant.' There was no response so she kept talking, changing the subject to say that Dad was here and Leasa and Darren and Ryan and they had a little flat around the back of the hospital so they could stay close to him. He looked at her as if he understood but then he slept and when he woke up he didn't know what she was on about.

'What flat?'

So she told him all over again. Every morning by about eight o'clock she was at his bedside. 'I wanted to be there. I wanted to learn everything, even how to say these drugs that I couldn't say the name of.'

There was a lot to learn. Marc struggled to understand what had happened. As the sedatives began to wear off he felt pain all over his body, although weirdly he said he also felt stronger. Whenever anyone mentioned the heart transplant he went very quiet, as if he was frightened to think about that. Linda wanted to know everything though, she devoured the information from the nurses. Marc's breastbone had been broken open then bound together with wire, which would be there for the rest of his life. Tubes in his chest would stay for a few days to drain away fluid that could otherwise fill up his lungs and cause him to drown and he was still being fed through the nose. There were other tubes into his body that Linda didn't understand at all.

Now she was told her son would need to take drugs to suppress his own immune system. This had tried to save his life by fighting the virus when it first attacked him but now it wanted to repel another invader: his new heart. If that should happen, he might complain of chills or a fever, palpitations in his chest or extreme fatigue. The doctors didn't say how on earth he was supposed to identify any of that when he was already under heavy sedation and in all kinds of discomfort, but they did say that the immunosuppressant drugs that were his defence against the body rejecting the heart also came with nasty side effects.

Cyclosporine could make him sick, give him the runs or the shakes or send his blood pressure zooming up. Prednisolone could make his skin thin and crack, weaken his bones and fatten his face. Others might lead to muscle cramps or really sore joints. All of them could harm him but they were also going to keep him alive.

'This lovely nurse sat with me and tried to tell me how to pronounce the drugs but she was doing it all in a Geordie accent, I just couldn't get it.'

Broad Scots met broad Geordie in a clash of vowels.

'Sy … clo … spor … un …'

'Say that again?'

The nurses suggested she keep a record of which medicine was taken when, because there was so much to remember. The first batch of drugs could weaken his bones and push up his blood pressure, so he had to take more drugs to resist both of those. Then there were even more drugs to stop his body retaining water, reduce the risk of blood clots and fight infection. They would check his progress by carrying out a heart biopsy, which meant threading a tiny grab through a vein in his neck and into the heart to snick out a sample of the tissue there. That would show warning signs if the heart was being rejected.

Thankfully, there were none.

A professor who came to see Linda said: 'What happened to Marc was one in forty million. I've never seen anyone survive who was so ill, attached to so many machines with every organ failing. It's a miracle he is here.'

When he was awake, struggling with the pain and discomfort and his fear of what was going on, Marc suddenly had a really vicious temper on him that Linda had never seen before. He shouted at his mum, swearing at the top of his voice when she didn't act fast enough to press the buzzer to tell the nurse he was having another attack of diarrhoea, a side effect of the drugs. 'Just get out of my face!'

Linda ran off to the kitchen, where the nurse came and found her. 'Are you okay?'

'He's shouting at me, swearing. I don't get it. He doesn't do that, my Marc.'

'Listen – that's a good thing, Linda. He's not taking this lying down. He's angry and he wants to fight back. It's hard for you, but it's a great sign. Think of it like that, yeah?'

Linda was glad she was there. Grateful, too, that Marc had been unconscious and missed so much of the drama. She fought her own instincts and tried not to tell him too much more about what had happened while he was unconscious, in case he got confused or distressed. 'Marc never went through all the grief that we did. He never actually saw what was going on.' The downside of that was he struggled to understand how much his life was going to have to change. 'He was a young boy, he was a teenager, and now we were all saying, "Right, Marc, you've been a big healthy, fit boy but now you've got someone else's heart and you've got to take all these drugs for the rest of your life." It was a hell of a lot to take in.'

TWENTY-ONE

MARTIN

There would be no Christmas tree in the Burton home that year. Normally Nigel put it up in the lounge and hung out the lights for Sue and Martin to decorate the tree, but Martin wasn't there and the festive season was a hard reminder of his absence, coming only a few months after the funeral. 'You always think your son is going to grow up, fall in love and get married. Hopefully, they'll give you grandchildren. They'll bring the kids round and you'll have a nice, happy family Christmas all together,' says Nigel. 'There was a shock realisation at that time, all over again. You've lost all that, it's gone. He's never going to get married, he's never going to come round with the grandchildren. It's not just your loss, you feel sorry for him that he's never going to have all that now.'

Christopher was not interested in hanging shiny baubles, he was grieving in his own fierce way, says Sue. 'When we committed the ashes in the Garden of Remembrance he was saying, "How many times are we going to say goodbye?" I understand that. I think you never completely feel like you've said goodbye. I still don't now.' It would be many years before the Burtons put up a tree again, and that was for their first grandchild. Back then, nobody felt like celebrating that first Christmas. Martin's room was still as he had left it. 'He had these disgusting trousers that he wore all the time. The bottoms were all ragged. They were on the washing line, on the whirligig outside when we got home. I ripped them off the line and threw them in the bin. That's the anger of early grief. I could have quite happily gone into Martin's room, ripped everything down that reminded me of him, and got rid of it. Thankfully, I didn't. There was going to be a time I would treasure those things. I did the opposite, which was to just shut the door on it all. I couldn't deal with it.'

She had managed to go back to work, with the support of her boss at the small partnership of solicitors, who told her: 'Come back at your own pace. If you get up one morning and you can't face it, don't come in. If you get here and you're struggling, go home.' Sue knew that she had to do this. 'I needed some sort of structure in my life. That's just me. I also knew that if I didn't go back then I might never do it. I could still say it hurts too much. Every day of my life. So even if I had waited six months, I would still have had to face them all eventually.'

On her way to the office one day she saw a boy up ahead on a bicycle in the uniform of Martin's school. From behind, he looked just like her son. For a moment – a terrible, ripping raw moment – she thought it was him.

'It was ridiculous. I knew it couldn't be. But for a second, that boy was Martin.'

Sue cried all the way to work and cried some more when she got there. There were other triggers for her feelings too. It might be a case she was working on or something that somebody said in the office that set her off.

'I'd just put down my pen and go. Get out.'

Half an hour later, she'd come back to her concerned colleagues.

'You all right? Do you want a cup of tea?'

They learned to let her cry, or sit quietly, and in a while she would recover. 'If I want to go home, I'll tell you,' she said. But mostly she stayed. It was good to work, even if going on with normal life sometimes felt like a betrayal. 'The bills keep coming, so you have to work. The family needs feeding, so you have to go to the shops. You buy some bread and milk and you put the bins out. All those things you don't want to do, because they are too normal. By doing something normal, you are accepting what has happened. This is the new normal. You don't want to accept that, you really don't. But the bins still need putting out.'

Sue got caught out again when she was shopping in Asda. The supermarket tannoy started playing 'The Tide is High' by Atomic Kitten, the tune from Martin's funeral. She froze at first, then ran.

'I had a trolley full of shopping but I just left it and got out of there as fast as I could. That song still stops me in my tracks, even now.'

At least Sue and Nigel had each other. They were strong together, having been partners for a long time. They had both grown up in the same village outside Lincoln and been part of a gang of friends who went to school on the same bus every day, until he left to join the Royal Air Force at seventeen.

'I was stationed at a base nearby and I needed someone to go to a dance with me and I didn't have a girlfriend at the time, so I asked Sue. I didn't have to take a girl, but it helps if you want to dance,' he says, drily. 'That's how it started and we went from there.'

Sue was only sixteen when they danced, but she knew what she wanted and it was him. They got engaged as soon as she turned eighteen and were married in 1980. She quickly discovered the reality of being an RAF wife, which was that her husband would be away for long spells abroad. Even when he was stationed in this country, he would often have to be away during the week and only come home at weekends. 'It's not an easy life. We spent more of our marriage years apart than we did together. That's probably why we're still together …'

Christopher was born in 1983, after a terrible labour. Sue forgot it well enough to have another go four years later and this time the baby was born so quickly he was blue. She wondered about that when she was casting back for reasons for his death. She thought about the measles he suffered as a baby and the drugs she had taken to stave off nasty sickness all through the pregnancy. She even thought about the time Martin fell off his skateboard at the age of eight and bumped his head. All these things would churn inside her in her grief, but they were a happy family when the boys were young, even though Nigel was away a lot.

He was sent to Belize to look after Puma helicopters at an army training camp when Martin was only eight months old. 'You have to remember, there were no mobiles and no FaceTime. It was a phone call once a week from a phone box and that was it.' Sue learned to keep her feelings to herself during those calls. 'The last thing he needed was me whinging down the phone, saying, "I can't cope without you, when are you coming home?" As a Forces wife, you can't be like that. You have to cope.'

Nigel also developed the ability to just get on with things. 'You have to switch off from that and work. You can't worry about what is going on at home. If you stew on it too much it will wreck you.'

Holidays became very important, but they were all on holiday together at a caravan park in Scarborough when Saddam Hussein invaded Kuwait in 1990 and Nigel had to go. He was called out to the Middle East for the first Gulf War, to look after Tornado fighter bombers. 'Nobody joins the air force because they want to fight a war. My father was in the RAF as a radar technician and I joined because I wanted to work on aircraft, it was as simple as that. I accepted that if military force was needed by our country I was going to have to be part of that. You have to deal with it the best way you can.'

Sue was left with the boys, who got on well. 'They were far enough apart in age that they didn't want to steal each other's toys. Christopher was very laid-back and just accepted everything Martin did. Martin was like me, extremely short-tempered, but Christopher could handle him and they had a lot of laughs together.

Martin would get back from school earlier because he was that bit younger and he'd always want his big brother so you'd hear Chris shouting: "Get out of my room!" After we lost Martin, he said that was one of the things he missed. His little brother in his doorway, yacking away. The things that have driven you mad are often the things you miss the most.'

TWENTY-TWO

MARC

Marc felt like he had been smashed to pieces and glued back together the wrong way, but there was no escape from the physiotherapist. She came to see him every day, at first encouraging Marc to sit up a little, then a few days later to sit up properly and after a week or so even to dare to put his feet on the floor and try to stand. He felt sick and dizzy immediately and had to lie back down, head thumping. But the next day she came again, and challenged him to try again. He felt sick again, but not as much as before. And the day after that, when she brought a friend to help her help him, Marc stood up properly for the first time. The strong legs that had made him such a great football player were now weak and he was thin, laughably thin, having lost three stone since he fell ill.

'You're like a cowboy,' said his mum, trying to cheer him up.

'What you on about?'

'Look at you!'

It was true. As Marc began to take his first steps, then walk as far as the end of the bed, then to the door of the room, it became obvious he was lopsided now. The stroke had given him a curious swagger, like a sheriff walking down Main Street at High Noon. But he was a cowboy with no hope of jumping on a horse any time soon, who had to carry a little box with him when he walked. It looked like a silver PlayStation but the wires coming out of it went under his shirt and under his skin, right into his heart. The electrical pulse sent from inside the box kept his heart rate constant.

'What's this then, a hotel?'

Norrie was surprised when he came to see his son in the adult ward. This was late September, almost a month after Marc had first been rushed to hospital and he had passed his sixteenth birthday now, so he was no longer with the children. The rooms here were organised along a corridor and all made out in dark pine, which gave the place the feel of a Swedish lodge. His cubicle had a bed, an armchair by the window and a bedside cabinet and all was far less clinical than before, although the nurses were still in and out constantly. Lynne Holt had an office nearby and she was keeping an eye on the McCays, knowing that the days after the transplant can be difficult for everyone, as they try to understand the new normal. Families react in all sorts of ways. One man whose wife sadly died following a heart transplant asked for her old heart to be put back into her body for the burial, in place of the new one that had been rejected. 'We still had the heart, it was in the lab. We are very careful about the way we handle organs these days. I hope it gave him some peace.'

Then there was the mother who lost her baby child after a transplant and asked to be given the original heart to take home. 'I was worried about that, but after talking to her I said, "Would you like to see the heart, to say goodbye?"' She left the mother in a room with the heart, which was in a see-through plastic bag in a white pot, a bit like a beach bucket. Lynne opened the bag and rolled the edges back. 'I don't know what she did in there, or whether she touched the heart, but I do know that when she came out she said, "Thank you." That was enough for her.'

The patients had to be watched closely too. Some felt revulsion towards the organ that had been put inside them, but that was rare. Others believed they were beginning to think and feel differently, taking on the thoughts and emotions of the person whose heart they had received, although they usually knew very little about them.

This may not have been so strange, actually. Science is beginning to explore the idea that the heart doesn't just receive signals from the brain telling it what to do, it also sometimes ignores those instructions and sometimes sends back its own messages. We seem to have something called system memory, allowing organs to store information, which would make a little sense of some of the more extraordinary accounts given by transplant patients like Claire Sylvia, a dancer and choreographer who had a heart and lung transplant in the late Eighties and said she found herself strutting like a young man, craving beer and chicken nuggets from KFC. Her donor was an eighteen-year-old man who liked these things far more than she did. Then there were the American patients interviewed for an academic study the year before Marc's operation. A college professor reported seeing flashes of light in his face all the time, then his donor turned out to be a police officer shot in the face while trying to arrest a drug dealer. A man who received the heart of a seventeen-year-old music student and violinist found himself strangely drawn to classical music. A very macho man was given the heart of a woman and started wearing a lot of pink and putting on perfumes he had never even let his wife wear. Some of this could be put down to coincidence, said the study, but not all of it.

An eighteen-year-old called Danielle was shown a photograph of the boy whose heart she had received after his death in a car crash. She was told he had written songs before his death including one called – incredibly – 'Danny, My Heart is Yours'. The response recorded by the researchers was powerful. 'I knew him directly. I would have picked him out anywhere. He's in me. I know he is in me and he is in love with me. He was always my lover, maybe in another time somewhere. How could he know years before he died that he would die and give his heart to me? How would he know my name is Danielle? His song is in me. I feel it a lot at night and it's like he is serenading me.'

The families of the people who give their hearts and the people who receive them are usually kept apart, and direct contact between them almost never happens. It could get very complicated. But Marc McCay was not prone to rushes of emotion, as he told a psychologist when she came to see if he was feeling okay.

'Aye, I am, thanks, no bother.'

He was not the sort to be fazed by a massive, life-threatening illness, a possible near-death experience and the most invasive surgery known to humanity. Sometimes Marc was so laid-back it was as if he barely knew what was going on. Then again, his mum would catch him in quiet moments with his hand on the dressing on the wound in his chest, trying to take in all that had happened to him.

Marc was fit enough to be discharged from the ward a month after the operation as long as he lived in the transplant flat. It was a place on the hospital estate where he could stay independently but see the doctors, nurses and therapists every day. His big sister Leasa spent a lot of time with him in Newcastle then, pushing him to the park near the hospital in his wheelchair and helping him to walk again or just hanging out. They became close, and she was able to ask what it had been like for him, to be in so much trouble.

Marc smiled. 'I just fell asleep, then I woke up again.'

'And how do you feel, you know, about getting a heart from someone?'

'I'm just happy that I'm here.'

That's how he was. As he became more alert, less druggy, he noticed that one of the nurses was cute. She was pretty and had a nice smile, but he was a child in her eyes, so that was a bit of a blow. And it's hard to make a good impression with someone who has brushed your teeth while you're in a coma. But a surprise visit one day lifted his spirits.

'I wonder what your pals Donny and Franny are doing the now?'

'Aye, Dad, I know.'

'Be all right if they were down here now, wouldn't it?'

'Oh aye, it'd be good.'

Norrie laughed, and stepped outside the room. 'Next thing, the two of them dived in to see Marc. They'd been waiting there. You should have seen his face. Those boys stayed for days. You could see they were so close, it was great.'

His younger brother Daryl was eventually allowed to visit, aged just fourteen, and was not too alarmed. 'Marc was up in the flat and not in the ward. There were no tubes or anything on him. He just looked like he had lost a bit of weight. He showed me the scar on his chest. Everything was just light and easy, dead calm.'

Daryl had been left at home through all the drama, as the family tried to shield him from the worst of it. 'I stayed with my Nana. She was dead caring, like my best pal, my second mum. She wanted to tell me stuff but she thought I was too young to have the full situation explained to me. I had been in hospital myself when I was little so I just thought you went off there and got fixed and then everything was all right, because that's how it was for me.' He found his grand-mother crying in the kitchen after visiting Marc, but told her not to worry. 'It didn't register with me that he could die.'

Linda was worried about Marc, of course. She tried to compensate by taking charge of his care, perhaps a little too much sometimes. 'We were getting teaching from the nurses, to stop infection. I mean, things like, "Don't keep Mark's toothbrush in the bathroom, germs can sit on the surface of your toilet pan." That's how delicate it was for him. We would never be able to have pets in the house again, because animals can carry germs which could kill Marc.'

She felt safe at the Freeman Hospital. 'They were fabulous, they tell you like it is there. They were saying, "This thing could happen to Marc, but if it does we will treat it with this …" Absolutely brilliant, they knew what they were doing. If we had to pay for medical care, I dread to think how much I would owe the government, honestly.'

After four months in hospital it was time for Marc to go home, but Linda got scared. 'I was very frightened. They had support groups in Newcastle but I was going to be a couple of hundred miles away in Scotland with a sixteen-year-old son who had been through a heart transplant with all these drugs, all this terminology that was completely alien to us. What should we let him do? What should we not let him do? Who was going to help us at home? I just didn't know what we were going to do.'

The consultant actually suggested they move to Newcastle, but Linda said it was impossible. 'That wouldn't have been any good for Marc. He was a home bird, he loved Lochwinnoch and all his friends. He wanted to see his sister and his brothers on a daily basis.'

There was something else, too. The 'Get Well' cards had been joined by others offering congratulations. People seemed to think his struggles were over, but that just wasn't true. 'Transplantation is not a cure – it is the swapping of a life-threatening scenario for a medically-managed condition,' says the Children's Heart Foundation in its advice to families. 'In fact, you will be realising that medical intervention will go on throughout the child's life and that his or her future is uncertain.'

Marc would be home in time for Christmas but he was still very much in danger. One transplant patient in ten dies within a year of getting a new heart. There's only a fifty:fifty chance of surviving for a decade and after that the odds get a bit hazy, although they are slightly better for young people. But then every day is a bonus, that's what you're meant to say. 'Concentrate

on the positive,' said the ward psychologist, but Marc
didn't need telling. He just wanted to get on with his
life, get better and have a good time again … however
many Christmases he had left.

TWENTY-THREE

MARTIN

W hy did Martin die? As the New Year began and life calmed down, that question began to haunt Sue and Nigel. There was only one person who could give them an answer but he was a very busy man, in a hospital they never wanted to see again. Harish Vyas understood that, so he offered to come to them. The lead consultant for a hard-pressed children's intensive care unit does not usually have time for home visits, but Dr Vyas was an unusual man with a son of the same age and he could imagine some of what they were going through. He picked up a nurse from the hospital who specialised in helping bereaved families and they drove across to Grantham to face questions from Nigel, and first from Sue. 'Did Martin get this because he had measles as a baby? Was it because of the drugs I had to take for sickness when I was pregnant with him?'

'No, it's nothing to do with either of those things.'

Sue took some convincing. 'If there's nobody else to blame then you blame yourself. That's how mother-hood works. "I made him, it's my fault."'

Nigel wanted to know if there would have been any signs. 'Did we miss something?'

'There is nothing you could have done,' said Dr Vyas. 'Absolutely not. None of this is your fault. We now know for sure that he had a condition called Arteriovenous Malformation of the brain. There was no way of guessing it was there. Some people have headaches or seizures, which can be treated and are a clue. Other people live their whole lives without ever knowing what is happening in their head. Martin could have lived to be eighty and never had a bleed or it could have happened to him as a baby.'

There was no good reason for Martin's death at all then. It was just bad luck. Awful, unthinkable, hide-ous luck. The Burtons began to understand that more fully as the conversation went on. The bleed was not the result of a blow to the head when he fell out of bed, or anything else. Their son had been born with a problem nobody could see, sitting there silently all his life: a snag in the system that sends blood to the brain. A blemish like a birthmark. The blood coming up through an artery is meant to flow into a patch in the brain called a capillary bed, which will take the oxygen away, but in his case – in one, tiny instance – the bed just wasn't there. The artery connected directly to a vein, which should never happen. It was a tangle, an unfortunate mess. For years it sat there, silently. The blood pressure built up where the artery met the vein, but still Martin felt nothing. Then the blood vessels suddenly burst in the early hours of the morning, said Dr Vyas.

'It's like a twig snapping.'

Sue still remembered the deserted hospital. 'What if he had been taken to a decent hospital straight away, where they had specialist doctors? Grantham is tiny. Did he die because we live near a small hospital?'

Again, Dr Vyas said 'no' to Sue's questions, gently but firmly. 'The bleed was so massive that it was unlikely he was ever going to survive.'

The Burtons were slowly persuaded, says Nigel. 'You felt the doctor's compassion. His understanding. We were grateful for what he had to say.'

Sue agrees: 'He convinced me that the things I was worried about were irrelevant. Martin was born with this condition. Where we lived made no difference, it just all happened so quickly. I did need convincing of that.'

There was something else on their mind, though. What about Christopher? Could this happen to him?

They were terrified of losing their other son, and he was scared too. Harish Vyas remembers that he could sense how frightened they were, so again he did something unusual to try to help them. 'Statistically, it is very unlikely that Christopher would have had any problems but we organised an MRI scan on him, the results of which came out as completely normal. That reduced the amount of anxiety and unhappiness they were living with.'

The Burtons didn't ask this, but what could the doctors actually have done if they had found something wrong in Christopher's brain? 'That is a very interesting question. If you interfere with the blood supply in the brain you can end up with a massive stroke. And if the problem is in what we call 'tiger country', where surgery would cause more harm than good, well then, where does that leave us? I really don't know.'

As Dr Vyas remembers the conversation they had, he begins to look quite sad. 'I do feel very emotional about this. It is not something I can look at dispassionately, because it is somebody's child we are talking about and in this case that child died. It doesn't stop me being professional and objective about clinical management, but as I said to Nigel at the time in the ward, as they were taking Martin to theatre, the day I stop thinking about the patient as another human being with a family that is going through grief is the day I ought to stop working. Really.'

There was another, very private reason why Harish Vyas cared so much about this case. It was not just that he had a son of the same age as Martin, but also that he had made a promise a long time before, to a man he loved and admired more than anybody else in the world. He doesn't talk about it often, but that promise was made in a way that resonates with all that is to come.

Harish qualified at Guy's Hospital in London in 1975 and soon after that his grandfather came to visit from Kenya. Shambhu was a large, gregarious man who was also now very ill and he had come to England to see his grandson for the last time. He made it clear that these were their final days together, then asked this boy he loved so much to make a vow: 'Promise to me that you will never be corrupted in medicine.'

Harish was taken by surprise. It was a strange request, although he knew his grandfather had come across doctors in Kenya who were corrupt. Those who could afford medicine were treated well, while those who could not were left to suffer. Shambhu had organised, argued, campaigned and cajoled on behalf of the poor and set up charities to help them. Now that his grandson was in a land where everyone had the right to treatment for free from the cradle to the grave, Shambhu wanted him to swear that he would play a full part in that wonderful enterprise. 'Of course I will,' said Harish lightly, thinking it all a bit silly, but his grandfather heard his tone, looked at his expression and frowned.

'Don't be flippant, please. You have a great gift. Commit yourself to serving your patients.'

'I will.'

Then the old man took his hand and made him seal the promise in a way that stayed with Harish for the rest of his career. He thought of it every time he looked at a photograph of Shambhu on his desk or on his wall wherever and whenever he went to work. If his hours as a junior doctor were long and wearying and the hospital work was intense, distressing or traumatic, he would look at the image of his grandfather and remember the promise. Then he'd feel his shoulders go back, his chest fill and his head clear. 'There were times when I felt sorry for myself but I would look at him and think, "No, I'm all right. Get on with it." He was my absolute hero.'

His research was into the first breath a baby takes after being born. As Harish hung around maternity wards like an anxious father, he noticed a lovely young Scottish nursing sister called Catherine. As they became friends, then lovers, he told her about his grandfather. She understood that his patients came first, however hard it was to live with sometimes. 'All doctors married nursing sisters in those days. They were the only females you ever met when you were working all the time,' says Harish with a smile, knowing full well how unromantic that sounds. Then he adds, with feeling: 'It's hard to imagine how I could have functioned without her.'

They had four sons together but Harish admits that he was often absent, particularly when he took over the paediatric intensive care unit in Nottingham in 1993. 'It was a unit that needed development.' For a while he was the only consultant there, so he would stay in the ward all day and all night and all the next day and the next night if necessary. 'I need very little sleep. I can go for a few days without going to bed, no problem.'

His wife would bring in food for him. Once, in an effort to spend more time with one of his sons, he promised a day out in Nottingham if they could just pop into the hospital first, to see a patient. Just for an hour, he said. No more than that. The boy, who was nine years old at the time, was happy to sit in his dad's office and wait. But there was a crisis on the ward, another sick child needed care and the doctor became engrossed. When Harish looked up from his work, he realised it was past eleven at night and his own son had been forgotten all that time, abandoned in the office without anything at all to eat or drink. 'I rushed back and he was there, absolutely still, looking miserable. Very dry and very hungry. I could not apologise enough. The trouble is that when there is a sick patient who needs to be seen, you forget everything else.'

The boy forgave him, eventually. They all did, when they were grown men. 'I've lived with that guilt for many years. Now I have had absolution from my children.'

With age, Harish has become the spitting image of the man who inspired him to become the kind of doctor who would spend so much time and energy caring for Martin Burton and his family even after death. 'Every morning I look in the mirror and I see my grandfather.' And there is something more to say about the moment when his grandfather made him vow to stay true to his calling and care for his patients first, all those years ago; something that will echo through this story. The old man took his hand and asked again: 'Do you promise?'

Then Shambhu pulled his grandson's hand towards him, unfurled the fingers, and put the palm up against his own chest. Harish repeated the words, this time with his hand over his grandfather's heart.

'I promise.'

* * *

There is one thing the Burtons never asked, because in their shock and grief they accepted how things were done, and it is hard for the doctor to answer even now. When exactly did Martin die? Questions like that were easier in the old days. People were considered to have died when their heart stopped beating. That was that. By those old standards, Martin was still alive when they took him to the operating theatre and stopped his heart with potassium before removing it. The heart would have stopped naturally if they had just turned the ventilator off, because he could not breathe on his own, but it would have been too damaged to use. In the early days of transplants, a doctor in America was sued by a family for taking a heart before the machines were turned off but they lost and the law was changed. Now, it is clearly perfectly legal to do so in America if the brain is no longer working.

In Britain, we are even more specific: death has occurred when the brain stem has stopped functioning. That means the heart and lungs are not getting the signals to beat and breathe and the body will just shut down without mechanical help. Dr Vyas and his colleague did all the proper tests on Martin and were quite sure that was the case. 'Legally, Martin was dead when we did the first brain stem test.'

This was recorded as the time of death and the Burtons accepted that but it is not actually when

Martin died – only when the doctors were able to confirm that he had. So the question remains, then: at what point in time between his collapse in Sue's bedroom and the results of those hospital tests did Martin actually die? Dr Vyas pauses to think, because he wasn't in the ambulance or at Grantham Hospital in the middle of the night, although he has seen the records. 'There was intervention. Things like breathing and blood pressure were being manipulated as soon as he got to the first hospital, so it is hard to say. He had a catastrophic bleed at home and the brain continued to die slowly. I can say though that if his mother had not heard him that night she would have found him in the morning dead.' So the truth is that nobody really knows the answer, although he says there is one piece of evidence that suggests Martin was brain dead when he hit the floor of Sue's bedroom: the snoring. The deep, guttural sound was a sign that his swelling brain had dropped into the spinal cavity, cutting off its own blood supply and partially blocking his breathing. Just to be sure then, in the doctor's opinion, was there anything anybody could have done at any point that would have saved him?

'No, there was not. I don't think it was salvageable. We should be clear about that. Martin had no chance of survival. None at all.'

TWENTY-FOUR

MARC

M arc tried to get on with his life as the New Year began, but his mum struggled with that. It was still only five months since Linda had thought she had lost him forever. She had fought with all her strength to keep it together in the hospital and plead, cajole or persuade – or sometimes just damn well demand – that the doctors did everything possible and she couldn't just leave him alone now, thinking: 'Free-man's have done all this wonderful work to save my son, I need to take over here.' So she did that, with the very best intentions, but Linda now admits she took it all too far. 'I smothered him, that's the word. I remem-ber buying all these plastic tubs and sitting there fixing his medication for the day ahead. I didn't realise this for quite a while but my whole conversation with him would be, "Marc, have you taken your pills? What time is your next appointment?" I forgot how to enjoy life and spend time with my son. That wasn't the life he wanted either, to have me interfering with him all the time, but I was a nervous wreck. There was no help. Zilch. I could not sleep, I was up checking him all night, to see if he was breathing. It was worse than bringing your first newborn baby home.'

Her fear ran deep, as she confessed to her mother.

'Mum, they told me the heart is gonna last five or six years, what age will he be when he passes away? We're running out of time already.'

Wee tough Betty was having none of it.

'Linda, you better snap out of this, lady. What a terrible thing to think. That boy needs you, but he also needs you to let him live. You've got to let him enjoy life!'

His friends were a great help; they had all known each other since nursery school and came round often. When they could eventually go out together, with Marc at first in a wheelchair, they set the alarms on their phones to tell him when he should take his tablets. That was still not enough for Linda in her agitated state. 'I was worried constantly, phoning and texting him. I think he would turn his phone off just to get some peace.'

Sometimes, though, he did need her. Marc came through to her room at three in the morning with his quilt all wrapped around him and lay down on the bed.

'Mum, have you got any photographs of my great-grampa?'

'No, son. I never met that man. Are you okay?' There was a strange look on his face in the half light and he seemed shaken. 'What happened to you, Marc?'

'I had these dreams when I was under, Mum. I was looking out of this window and there was Leasa on the other side.'

Linda listened and made connections with what had happened in the hospital. 'You know what, that was the window in the high-dependency unit.'

'Then I was sucked down this pipe and all the faces changed.'

'Marc, that's when they were doing suction on you. There was a tube down your throat. You had two lungs collapse. The physios sucked all the gunk out. You must have been aware of that noise, to think you were getting sucked down that tube.'

'I saw this guy who said he was my great-grampa. Clear as I'm seeing you. We talked, then he said he had to let me go back. Then I woke up.'

Linda was stumped by that. She couldn't help him with any more information about the old man, but the next time Marc saw his dad he described what he had seen. Norrie dug out an old photograph and there he was, the man in the dream, looking exactly the same.

'Aye,' said Marc. 'That's the guy.'

What Marc did not know was that John McCay was originally from Ireland. He actually spoke with an Irish accent just like in the dream and pronounced his name to rhyme with eye, at least at first. When he fell for a young Protestant woman in tough, working-class Glasgow in the hard times of the 1930s, John found himself on the wrong side of the divide between Catholic and Protestant and the football clubs Celtic and Rangers. Not that he cared much, even when he found out her family were part of the staunchly Unionist Orange Order and didn't approve of him. There were frowns and threats but love won again and they got married anyway. To make life a little easier she made him say his name McCay to rhyme with hay, although quite how that was supposed to help has long been forgotten now, by Norrie at least, and he was the one with the information. His own formidable father – known to all as Mr McCay – was not one to share these things. 'You spoke when you were spoken to,' says Norrie, who rebelled against his dad. 'You did what he told you. Unless you could find a way not to …'

Norrie got a couple of Scottish symbols tattooed on his arms without permission when he was Marc's age and Mr McCay shouted at him: 'Next thing we know there'll be a lassie at the door and she'll be pregnant.' Norrie smiles at the memory and winks in recognition: 'He wasn't far off.' By the time he was thirty, Norrie was a father of five. 'I just had to look at Linda and she was pregnant.'

His granny, old John McCay's wife, had a soft spot for him and could make him laugh. 'She would say to me, "Norman! Are you sure that wee lassie's not a Catholic? I think she is, son!" You know, because of having all these kids? She was funny.'

Norrie freely admits he was never a romantic with Linda. 'See all that walking through the town holding hands with a lassie? That's not for me. I'd walk in front. Or behind even.' And what would Linda say to that? 'You're an unloving bastard.'

Still, there was no bad feeling after they divorced, he says. Nor was it awkward between them when they were in the hospital together in Newcastle, staying in the same flat.

Norrie's way of dealing with things was to go for a walk every now and then for a quiet cigarette outside. 'I like my own space. I knew we were in the right place in Newcastle. They had only given us a one per cent chance of getting there but Marc had made it, so I felt we'd come a long way and he was in safe hands.'

Then, when they all got back home, he tried to help Marc have some of his old life back, to give him a bit of hope and something to aim for. 'It was getting cold, coming on to winter, but we would take him down the football park in his wheelchair to watch games. It was freezing, but he was all wrapped up and it cheered him up. I just took it that Marc would get better. He'd had a wee blip in his life, now he was on his way back. I didn't think about how long he would have left, at all.'

TWENTY-FIVE

MARTIN

The card in Sue's hands took her breath away. Friends and family had all sent their love, sympathy and prayers but this was something different, a message from a stranger. 'It was spidery writing, very shaky. I remember thinking it was from someone either quite elderly or quite ill.' The card showed a tree of life rising from the ground with green leaves against a star-filled purple sky, and the words 'Thank You' in silver writing on the cover.

To whom it may concern,
I am very sorry for your sad loss. Thank you for
helping me to start to live my life again. It has made
such a lot of difference.
    Always grateful, Fred.

There was no other information, but that is the way with transplants, deliberately. The system is set up to protect people's privacy, not least because feelings are raw, says Nigel. 'Every time they have communication it reminds you of your loss, so people don't want to go there.'

Fred had written to the co-ordinator at his hospital, who had forwarded the card to their own transplant nurse in Nottingham and she had rung to ask if they wanted to read it. 'They promise you'll never get something in the post which you'll open up thinking it's something else and then go, "Agh!" It might hit you at a hard time, knock you for six on your way to work,' says Sue. 'You'll always know it's coming, they'll always give you that prior warning.'

The nurse also wrote with further news, but this time it was not so good. *'Unfortunately, the fifty-eight-year-old man who received a double lung transplant has since died. I am sure this must be upsetting for you to read and I am sorry.'* This must have been Fred. The card must have been sent before his death. *'This gentleman was terribly poorly prior to his transplantation, he received all possible treatment to try to improve his life, but unfortunately for his family this was not to be the case.'*

There was more. *'The lady that received a kidney transplant unfortunately had to have it taken out again as her body rejected the kidney.'* The doctors had taken every possible precaution, but her immune system had still refused to accept the organ. The gentleman who had been given the other kidney was doing well though, and is able to enjoy being with his grand-daughter for a while longer than he had feared.

'I am sure you are probably feeling exhausted reading this letter,' wrote the nurse, who offered to come and see them to talk things through. She did have some good news. *'The thirty-four-year-old gentleman that received a liver transplant continues to do well. He was suffering from a very rare condition that was extremely difficult to manage. He is now able to spend time with his two small children.'*

And the boy who had received the heart had now turned sixteen and was doing very well, she wrote. *'This boy was desperately ill prior to his transplant and would not have survived without it. Martin has had an incredible impact on this boy's life.'*

That was very true. They were bound together now in a remarkable way. But the impact Martin would have on Marc was not over yet. Not by a long, long way.

TWENTY-SIX

MARC

Linda loved her job at the Royal Alexandra Hospital and there were bills to pay, so when Marc was settled at home again in the spring she went back to work. Now, though, she found that everything had changed in her head. 'I was in a state. It was too close to home. The first night, a man passed away in Room 10. I went into the kitchen and I was sobbing, uncontrollably. I couldn't do my job any more. I tried but I kept going into tears.'

She went back again for the next shift and the next, hoping these feelings would somehow pass, but they got worse. Then Linda was moved to a different ward and had to go around the patients in the dead of night checking catheters. They were all asleep, the lights were low. She came to the end of the round and found herself standing outside the doors to Room 25. This was the high dependency unit, where Marc had been taken that first night, straight after she had blocked the ambulance bay and demanded to be seen. The fear came flooding back.

'I could hear the do-do-do of the heart monitor on a patient behind those doors. I swear to God I stood there frozen and the tears just came. This nurse came up and said, "Linda you're having a wee flashback. Come away with me, hen, and let's sort you out." We sat and had a cup of tea and I kept saying, "What am I doing here at work? I should be with Marc."'

Still she kept going, until the hospital extended the length of the shifts so she had to work twelve hours at a time, which was far too long for her to be away from Marc. Then she thought, 'It's not worth it.' But before she left, there was something she needed her friends at the hospital to help her do. Linda wanted to write to the family of the boy that had given Marc his new heart, whoever they were, to say thank you. 'I had this overwhelming urge to let them know how grateful we were and how much their son was loved for what he had done. His heart had not just saved Marc, it had saved my other three sons, my daughter, everybody in the whole family. There was a ripple effect. We are very close, we see each other or speak every day and if we had lost Marc then I don't think my family would have recovered.'

The transplant nurses at the hospital said they would ask the donor family if they wanted to have anonymous contact. 'I used to drive the co-ordinator nuts, until eventually he was getting fed up with me and he said, "Okay, you can write a letter. Just say a few things about this and that, don't go on too much."'

So while she was still working at the Royal Alexandra in the summer of 2004, only six months after Marc's return home, four of her fellow nurses sat down together in the staffroom and helped Linda write the letter. It reads now like it was written by a committee of very caring people, well aware of the damage they would do if they got it wrong. 'We were all in floods of tears trying to get it right.'

TWENTY-SEVEN

MARTIN

Dear Friends,

First and foremost we would like to express our deepest condolences for the loss of your son. I would also like to apologise for any grief or upset this letter may cause you.

This is the most difficult letter I have ever had to write. I cannot begin to stress how your decisions, choices and emotions that you went through (which are unimaginable) are so much appreciated and the choice you made saved my son's life.

Our fifteen-year-old son, Marc, was the top goal scorer for his football team, a big, strong, healthy boy who had never been ill. Marc felt unwell on 20th August last year. Within days he was on a life support machine, a virus had attacked his heart and twice we were told he was dying of uncontrollable heart failure and multiple organ failure. In order for Marc to have any chance he was to be transferred to Newcastle, where he was placed on a machine which would keep him alive temporarily, until a donor heart may or may not become available.

Marc had a 99 per cent chance of not making the journey.

All of the above took place and on 29th August 2003, Marc successfully came through a 12-hour operation. Unfortunately, in order for the heart transplant to take place that night, your son's life was lost.

Marc is doing remarkably well and hopefully has an illness-free life ahead of him. I thank God every day for your decision. My entire family could never express in any way or form our heart-felt thanks and deep gratitude.

My thoughts are with you every day and especially will be on 29th August.

Should it give you even a shred of comfort, please do not hesitate to contact us at any time.

Marc will be seventeen on 8th September and that has been made possible because of you. Thank you for your son's heart.

Linda McCay,

Marc's Mum

There was a card too, with a pink cover and a poem that began with the words, 'Angel of Love – Thank You'. Members of the family had signed it and given their relationship to Marc in brackets. There on the top left was his own signature too, Sue realised with a little shiver of surprise. Marc had put his name in friendly, curvy letters, not quite joined up, but under-lined. An almost childish hand, as Martin's would have been, and the message was a little playful. 'Thinking of youz ALWAYS.'

This was him. He wrote this, thought Sue, imagin-ing a pen in a teenage fist. Then a slip of paper fell out of the package and it was a newspaper cutting, thin in her fingers, with the headline: 'Heart transplant gives brave teen Marc a second chance at life'. His face stared up from the paper, straight at her. A very hand-some young man in a red and white football kit with his hair razored at the side but spiky on top. Well, he probably wanted it to be spiky but it was fluffy, really. Marc was frowning and looking into the camera with a cocky half-smile, as you might when you're a lad having your picture taken as part of a team, maybe to celebrate a big win. His portrait had been cropped from a larger image, it was blurry but Sue still had a strong sense of him, for the first time. There he was, a boy. A lad like her Martin, who loved his football. The kind of lad Martin might have liked to have been, all sporty and dashing, if he had been bothered about that sort of thing. They might have been friends, though. Mates. Marc looked just like one or two of the boys who had been at the funeral, that hair was the style they had.

She sat down and went on staring at the image as the paper clipping trembled slightly in her hand. Marc stared back. He was real suddenly, not an idea or a name on a list but a real person, this person, going about his business, living his life, playing his sport, with Martin's heart inside him. Something about that disturbed Sue and frightened her. Something about it was a little bit comforting, somewhere deep inside.

'That was a nice moment, because I could put a face to him. We knew he had suffered a sudden illness and needed a heart very urgently, but up until then he was just this faceless person. Now I could see him. It was good to see that this person did exist and to be told he was doing really well, but it was really odd to think of Martin's heart still beating inside him while he was walking and running around somewhere far away.'

So now she knew their names and where they lived. The McCays. It made a difference to her, a really big one. Alongside the loss and the grief and the anger there was now also the knowledge that somebody had been helped, somebody had a life because of Martin.

No, not just somebody in general, not any more. This person. This Marc, this good-looking chap. This Linda and all the other names on the card, which she couldn't quite take in. Sue was still at the point where it felt like a betrayal of her son to enjoy life without him, but she did feel their thanks like a rush of warmth, if only for a moment. So what now?

Sue was glad to get the letter but she could not reply immediately for fear of all the feelings it would stir up. She was working to stay away from those every day, for her own survival. It took her a few weeks to find the strength to write back and tell this Linda all about her Martin, mother to mother, enclosing a picture of her son, but she did want to do it. 'I wanted Linda to know that I was glad Marc was doing well. I didn't want her to think I was resentful of that, in any way. I was really grateful that she had taken the time to write to me, but I believed it would be a one-off thank-you and that would be all the contact we ever had. I didn't dream there would ever be such a strong bond between us.'

As the anniversary of her son's death approached, Sue was lonely in her grief. She needed to talk to someone who understood what she was feeling, because no friendship or marriage is ever strong enough to bear such a burden alone. 'We had some fantastic support from our friends, don't get me wrong, but everyone would say, "I can't imagine what you're going through." Or else other people would say they were really sorry and start talking about how they had lost their parents. I've lost both my mum and dad since I lost Martin and I can say without hesitation that there's a bloomin' big difference. I needed to have contact with people in the same situation.'

Help came from a charity called the Donor Family Network. Sue rang them and poured her heart out to someone who listened and it helped her get through. In time, she would become a volunteer herself. For now, she was having to make decisions now about what to do with Martin's room and his stuff and it was tough. 'If I had to go in that room I went in and out as fast as I could, for a long, long time. Then of course you get the complete turnaround, where actually going in that room is special, because there are memories in there. It might bring forth tears, but to be in with his things is very special. So you go from one extreme to the other, from not being able to cope even looking at something to actually wanting to hold their clothes, smell their clothes, it's their room, it's their things …'

She was also able to ask how other people had coped. 'I know people who've left everything in the bedroom, even the half-mouldy sandwich. We've never kept it as a shrine. We tidied it up and sorted it out. Martin had West Ham wallpaper and curtains and a duvet cover and I found that really hard to see. So it was a very conscious decision to decorate the room so that we could go in there without feeling the pain. It was that or just never open the door.'

They got rid of the bunk bed Martin slept in and replaced it with a double bed for Chris and his girl-friend. 'Chris only had the box room with a single bed. We didn't know how they'd feel about sleeping on a double bed in Martin's room but they said they would.'

Nigel and Sue cleared out Martin's room together, on their knees on the floor, sorting through stuff and talking about their memories. Together, they were able to be quite clear-headed about what they wanted and what could go. 'I know bereaved parents who've got every last thing of their child's possessions boxed up in the loft, never to be seen again, which to me personally seems a bit pointless. It would get stuck up there and left to the next person to deal with when we're gone, which would be Christopher, and that is unfair. I don't want to put that on him. So we did have a sort out and get rid of rubbish. I mean, a teenage boy's bedroom? I need say no more.'

Getting rid of his clothes was the hardest. 'I had numerous sessions where I'd open the wardrobe door, get them out and try and sort them. I'd sit on the floor and sob then put them all back again and shut the door. "Okay, never mind, we don't do that today then." I believed that I'd do it when I was ready.'

She found a clever, creative way to cope, eventually. 'I went on a support weekend for bereaved parents. Somebody brought along a quilt they had made using squares cut from their child's clothing, so I started my own quilt. That way you can keep little bits of lots of things without having this pile of clothes that nobody will ever wear. You end up with something beautiful.'

'How many years have you been making that quilt now?'

'Quite a while, Nigel. But I will finish it one day.'

The Burtons are organised people, that is one of their strengths. 'We've got a memory box. It's got some of Martin's school books in it, with his handwriting on. That's very special. It's got his cap, his watch, his school tie. Favourite bits and pieces I know I'll keep forever. I've also got his teddy sat on my bed.' They have a few good photographs but not as many as a family would have now, because smartphones with cameras were not everywhere in those days, says Sue. 'We've got nothing with his voice on. Not a thing. It's so hard. I can remember what he looked like, just like that, because I've got loads of pictures, but voices fade away in your memory. You think you can remember, but you can't. That is the one thing I would love to have, his voice.'

Then, as they faced the second anniversary of Martin's death, the Burtons received another letter from Nottingham. This time the transplant nurse was happy to give the first names of all of the surviving patients who had received organs from Martin and say that each one of them was recovering well. *'Marc was in the clinic a few weeks ago with his mum and is described as a bonny, blond lad, always happy.'*

They already knew that, of course, because of the letter from Linda.

'The kidney patient, Eric, is still fit and well and despite his age is continuing to work as a plumber. His kidney function is entirely normal and he feels great.'

The liver patient, Andrew, had to be seen often because of his unusual condition, but he was able to lead a relatively normal life. *'His disease means that he is extremely sensitive to light and therefore cannot play outdoors with his children. He has decided this year to book a holiday abroad in a villa with a swimming pool. This will allow his wife to play with the children during the day, but he will be able to swim with them in the evenings. He is so looking forward to this. It would have been impossible to have this sort of a holiday without the transplant.'*

That was the most Sue expected to hear from any of them. 'That's all the majority of donor families will ever get. We made it clear from the start that we were happy to have more contact but they said that sort of thing just didn't happen. You've got to be pretty sure that both parties are going to be able to deal with it emotionally. They wouldn't want us stalking people, demanding to know what they were doing all the time and saying, "You can't do that, it's not good for our heart."'

So that was that. They tried to move on with their lives, missing Martin every day of course and being snagged by grief at unexpected moments, but concentrating as much as they could on the future. Sue and Nigel went to help out with the Transplant Games, a competition run for those who have had life-changing surgery, but a conversation there made her think again. 'I was in the bar in the evening and got chatting to one of the dads. He was a bit over the top when he found out I was from a donor family and his wife asked if she could give me a hug. You tend to think, "Can't they just put pen to paper and say thank you?" I didn't understand how hard that was.'

The mother explained that she had often thought about writing to their donor's family through the nurses but couldn't find the words, because she was worried. 'How can I tell them that their decision has given me my daughter back? It will rub salt into their wound.'

Sue reacted strongly to that, telling her: 'It won't, you know. They made that decision at a time of tragedy that was going to happen anyway. They need to know some good has come out of it.'

She was taken aback by her own strong reaction and thought about it all the way home. She had already replied to Linda's letter but now decided to write via the transplant nurse to the other people who had been given organs from Martin, to say she was glad and proud he had been able to help them. 'I wanted to say, "We miss Martin every day, but we're glad we made the decision we did." I didn't expect to hear back.'

There were no contact details, of course, and no clues that would allow people to trace her – but by an extraordinary coincidence, one of the people who got the note was actually writing to her at exactly the same time. The transplant nurses who are usually so cautious saw that the letters had crossed and put them directly in touch. That was unheard of, but it happened in this case. It was the beginning of an unexpected relationship that would endure. Surprisingly, it was not with either Linda or Marc …

TWENTY-EIGHT

ANDREW

They call it Vampire's disease. You can't go out in direct sunlight or your skin blisters. You stick to the shadows or only dare to venture out at night. Your lips peel back and your gums may shrink, exposing the teeth so they look like fangs. Your skin is yellow, tightening on the skull with dark, sunken eyes. Your face may become disfigured and you could lose your ears or nose. You are not a monster, but the sight of men and women like you has struck fear into ignorant people throughout history, inspiring myths and legends about night-dwellers, bloodsuckers and vicious, demonic werewolves as well as the vampires who give the disease its horrible nickname.

The real name is porphyria, from the ancient Greek word for purple, because the urine of those afflicted turns the colour of port wine. Instead of being given medical help, many have been driven from their homes over the centuries, disowned or even burned at the stake.'

Andrew Seery was lucky enough to be born at a time when doctors had identified this as a genetic condition caused by too many porphyrins, chemicals in the body that exist to help produce a vital part of red blood cells. On the other hand, his childhood was troubled. His father was an alcoholic and his mother had a breakdown, so when he was nine years old Andrew was taken into care, where he was teased mercilessly because of the way he looked. 'I was always the boy that had scabs on his face from the burns, which were very painful. I always wore long sleeves and a hat and I used to always want to be in the shade. I would criss-cross the road to be out of the sun so it would take me much longer to get anywhere.'

Shunned by the other kids, he was about to commit suicide by throwing himself into a river at the age of twelve when he felt someone close by. 'An old man looked at me and shook his head. I was really scared because I knew I shouldn't have been doing this, so I bottled it.'

Instead of killing himself he started to pray and over time became a Christian, which he says helped him to survive. Andrew managed to cope with his condition enough to train as a hairdresser, fall in love, marry and have children; but as he grew older, the porphyria got much worse. 'My tolerance to sunlight deteriorated in my late twenties, until being outside was really painful. There was no cure for it. I kept going, but that summer of 2003 I was cutting hair at one of my two salons in Basingstoke when I started getting pains in my side. The next day I was yellow.'

The doctor said his liver was failing and asked how much he drank, but Andrew laughed. He barely drank at all. 'That was a dark moment, because if it had been the drink you could just cut down, couldn't you?'

After three weeks of uncertainty, growing weaker, he was sent to the specialist unit at Addenbrooke's Hospital in Cambridge for a bone marrow transplant, but when he got there they said he was too late. There was too much damage, his liver would not cope with the operation. By now, Andrew was close to death. 'I was down to six stone four, in a wheelchair, being fed on a nasal drip and very, very weak.'

They told him he needed a liver transplant but the waiting time was nine months. 'I didn't have nine months. They didn't think I would last anywhere near that long. I knew then that someone would have to die if I was going to be saved. That was weird. If I saw an ambulance before this, I would say a prayer for the people in it. Now I was thinking, "That could be my chance to live."'

Andrew was only thirty-four years old. His daughter was eight and his son was ten. 'When you have got children that age you become a little selfish. I prayed, "Lord, let me see them grow up." You don't wish anyone harm, but you have a great desire to live.'

Andrew went home to Winchester and spent most days in bed. 'If I got out of bed to make a cup of tea, that would be all I could do for the day, my energy would be gone. I was anxious, thinking each day was my last on the planet.'

The telephone rang in the early hours of the Friday morning in late August – when Martin was in the operating theatre, although Andrew knew nothing of that – and his wife took the call. A liver was available, it was being collected now. She drove him to Addenbrooke's as quickly as possible, which took nearly three hours as they had to get around the M25 and up the A1 in the early morning traffic. 'I went straight into theatre,' he says.

The surgeon Paul Gibbs operated in the dark because of Andrew's condition, working by ultraviolet light to take out his diseased liver and replace it with the healthy one from Martin. 'We had UV filters on all the theatre lights and with screens on the windows blocking out all natural light, so the theatre was very strange,' the doctor told a reporter afterwards. 'We had lots of people come in and say, "What on earth's going on in here?" because it was very dark apart from these pools of blue light around the anaesthetic area and the operation itself.'

This was such an unusual case that the surgeon talked to the *Guardian* about it afterwards. 'It's a complex procedure, both surgically and physiologically for the patient and therefore for the anaesthetist. When you don't have a liver you're not making a lot of the normal proteins and performing a lot of the homeostatic mechanisms that are necessary for life. And, depending on how you do the liver transplant, you might also cut off part of the blood supply back to the heart, so you might need to put them on to bypass. The anaesthetist needs to support them during that procedure. In some cases, where there has been a lot of bleeding, it's the anaesthetist who has a crucial role as much as the surgeon – it's a real team event to get the patient through.'

Mr Gibbs said he was in the darkened operating theatre for eight hours with his team. 'You get the liver out, put the new liver in, plumb the blood vessels into it, you get reasonable blood clotting achieved, then you go off and have lunch and leave it for half an hour for the anaesthetist to stabilise the patient and also for the new liver to start working. That's a useful period of time for the stabilisation of the patient as well as good for the surgical team to have a rest.'

Despite the strange conditions, they were relaxed. 'You don't go into an operation thinking if I do this wrong, this patient will die, because if you did that all the time you wouldn't be able to do it. You're talking to the anaesthetists, or to the other surgeons, about what you did yesterday or what you are doing at the weekend. If it's a difficult, concentratey bit, you concentrate and stop talking, and then you start talking again. It's very relaxed and there's lots of black humour.'

Andrew had been told his liver was coming from a teenage boy, but there were no other details. 'My first thought was, "Oh no!" I presumed it was a road accident, I didn't know then that they had to keep him alive on a machine for a while for me and the others, that's amazing.' Andrew had other things to worry about, as his body rejected the liver. 'I had loads of problems, including pneumonia. I'd go home for a week then have to go back. There was a problem at the point at which the liver was attached to me, the bile was going back up the pipe and it was all going wrong. A couple of weeks before Christmas they said I would have to have another transplant but I prayed about it and when I went back after Christmas the consultant said, "I don't know what you've been doing or eating but you are fifty per cent better."'

His recovery began to speed up. 'I was doing things I hadn't done for years. I used to poke my head out of the window when it was sunny and think, "Wow, I can feel the sun on my skin." It was great to be able to eat without stomach problems, too.'

By now he had been told the name of the young man who had given him this liver and he was talking to it. 'Mad, isn't it? You've got to cope somehow. If things were difficult I would say, "Come on, Martin, we've got to get through this." I still do talk to the liver, it does help, although if you think about it too much you could go over the top. There was one guy in hospital who totally flipped and tried to take his liver out, he was clawing at his body. I get a little wobble now and then, but I think, "It's not Martin. His soul has gone."'

That didn't stop him feeling survivor's guilt. 'You're alive and someone else isn't. When you believe that everybody is equal in the eyes of God and everyone has a right to life, it could probably bring you down, if you didn't find a way to handle it.'

His way of handling it was to try to get in touch with his donor's family: 'I would like to thank you in person.' He knew that was against the rules, so why suggest it? 'Writing a letter is not really good enough.

You can't say, "Thank you, I'm alive, your son's dead."
It was important to me to meet them.' The hospitals
usually consider that unwise, but in this case Sue
Burton had already written her letter to him and the
transplant co-ordinator said she had been waiting for
the right moment to pass it on: 'That's interesting, the
mother has been asking about you, too.'

They exchanged emails and Sue sent Andrew some
thoughts about her son's life and a photograph of
Martin. 'That was daunting. I looked on the computer
and saw his face for the first time. It wasn't a liver, it
was a person. I've had this sense of living two lives.
The fact he was so young inspired me to get the most
out of the time he had given me. You've got to live up
to the gift, be thankful instead of grumbling. Seeing
the face and reading about the life that had been
planned, it moved me. I did cry.'

His wife Geraldine was in the room with him when
the email came and she could feel his rush of sadness.

'Are you okay?'

'I'm not sure. Yeah. This makes it more real.'

Andrew insists that his liver ached when he saw
Martin. When he talks about it now, he reaches down
to put a hand on his side. 'I can feel extra activity in
the liver area, right now.'

* * *

Andrew is still skinny and sallow and he walks with a cane sometimes but he's better than he could have hoped, presiding over a crew of hairdressers in his salons, looking like Captain Jack Sparrow squeezed into a three-piece suit and trilby. He's a bit of a dandy with a silk square in his breast pocket, and as a lay preacher he likes to tell stories. 'We had this Geordie chef on the ward. One day he served steak and kidney pie and liver and onions. I'm not kidding. I had to say, "Are you having a laugh? This is a transplant hospital!" Seriously. Can you believe it?'

Andrew still has to have blood transfusions every week and they slow him down, but there's no doubt that he's loving his extra life. 'I'm not great in the morning, I puke up sometimes and I've lost my teeth, but that's cosmetic. I was never good-looking anyway. The liver has given me ten more years, now I've got to stay around to see the kids through university. My daughter wants me to walk her down the aisle someday, so no pressure! Children want your time, more than anything. They couldn't give a monkeys about flash holidays or a big house, they remember the ordinary things that cost nothing.'

He had to be careful about talking like that to Sue and Nigel when they came to visit him in Winchester, because of course they had lost their child. The *Guardian* had heard about the story and offered to put the

Burtons up in a hotel nearby for the night, but that meant there would be a camera present recording every moment, which made it awkward. 'I was still carrying a bit of guilt. Sue was in a bit of shock. I felt like she was looking through me to Martin. The next day she called me on the phone and said sorry. That was okay, it was hard for her. I told her there was nothing to apologise for.' Sue and Nigel had done him a great favour, by coming all the way down from Grantham and helping him not to feel bad about Martin's death, by saying they were only glad something good had come out of their tragedy. 'It made a massive difference to hear that from the parents, especially when you are a parent yourself. You sort of know that it's not your fault, but you don't know, deep down, as well. I'm not sure where the guilt comes from, but once I was cleared of it by that conversation, I just wanted to live.'

Andrew and Sue did meet again in time, and it was easier. Over the years they settled into a long-distance friendship, neither asking too much of the other, although he did anything he could to promote the cause of organ donation and help patients cope. 'I would say this to anyone who has had a transplant: don't settle for an ordinary life. Be the best you can be at whatever you do, find joy in that and if you can't then do something else. I will always be grateful to Nigel and Sue for releasing me from my guilt to be fully like I am now and live my life to the full.'

TWENTY-NINE

MARC

'I carried Sue's letter around with me everywhere I went and I kept getting it out, looking at this wee boy and crying,' says Linda, the mother of Marc. 'For about three months I did that, until my mother said, "You've got to stop this, hen." So I put the picture of Martin in my Bible. I don't go to church religiously, I don't read my Bible every day, but I do take what I want from it when I need to, whether that's reading Proverbs or the Psalms or whatever, so I put the picture in there. I would talk to him. I know that sounds cuckoo but I would thank him and say, "Your mum's brilliant." I didn't know anything about her but I felt I owed it to her to keep Martin's memory alive, his heart was beating inside Marc, that's the heart we were given.

'I asked Martin for help, too. I'd say, "If you're up there, please ask God to look after my Marc, don't let

Him take my son away from me after everything we have been through. You gave us this gift, Martin, I think it's your job to look after Marc."

'Some people think I'm mad, but it helps me to think about it like that. I did think of Sue all the time, as another mother like me, and I thought, "I would dearly like to meet you one day." I tried to find her many times over the years, on the Internet, but they didn't even give me her surname. I was pretty sure it was not ever going to happen, but I never gave up hope.'

Marc just wanted a normal life. If he was never going to be able to play football again then why couldn't he be like any other teenager and go out with the gang or stay up late for a poker game, drink whatever the hell he wanted and shake off the hangover in the morning? What was to stop him? His sister Leasa was torn between warning him not to put himself in danger and cheering his fight for the right to party. 'The doctors told us that as long as he took his pills at the right time, the only thing that was going to change in Marc's life was that he had to protect himself from the sun. He didn't need to have a restricted life. But he didn't need to kick the arse out of it, get mega drunk and sleep all the next day. He beat himself up over that later, but there is no way he should have blamed himself. It was a lot to put on a boy of sixteen.'

Football saved him. Out of the blue, as he got stronger, a cardiologist overturned the previous advice and told him to exercise as much as possible, to get the heart beating. So Marc stepped up the pace on the treadmill at the gym. He went to the local pool in Lochwinnoch and got fitter and fitter over the months, surprising himself. His confidence began to come back. He kicked a ball in the park and found that he hadn't lost his touch, although his chest would burn and his legs were quickly exhausted. Ultimately, he would play five-a-side with his brothers at the sports centre and then even join the village team for full games, although the coach was cautious.

'Marc, I'm not sure about this. We can't have you running about the park for ninety minutes. Maybe come on as a sub.'

'Aye, right,' said Marc, frustrated. 'I'll do that. For now …'

THIRTY

MARTIN

Real men don't cry. That's what they say, but it's rubbish. Nobody knows that better than Nigel Burton, who was trained in the armed services to keep his emotions in check, but found when he lost his son that it did him no good at all. 'Everybody expects the man to be strong, not to show emotion. The mum carries the child, gives birth to the child, there is always a very strong emotional psychological bond between a mother and a child and you have to accept that as a father, but society generally says the man should be the pillar of society, with a stiff upper lip. That is totally wrong. A lot of the men I have met who have lost their sons or their daughters say the same. Show your emotion. Do cry. Don't be afraid. You're just human and if you bottle it all up you will eventually break.'

Still, he was content to let Sue take the lead when it came to talking about their story in public, as she increasingly wanted to do as a way of dealing with the grief, to encourage others to sign up as donors. 'They always want to know about the mum anyway, the attention is all on the mother and not the dad. I'm happy with that. I understand.'

Sue was ready to tell her story to anyone who would listen, if it would help the cause. She was still very nervous when they asked her to appear on a television show called *The Big Questions* in February 2012. Sue would be sitting in the front row of a semi-circle as part of a panel talking about organ donation, with audience members behind her. Facing her was none other than Professor Richard Dawkins, the most outspoken scientist in the country, a champion of atheism with a habit of swatting away all those who disagreed with him. That was okay, though, she wasn't there to argue with him about God. She was going to tell the people in the room – and the couple of million people watching at home on a Sunday morning, although she didn't want to think about them – the story of Martin's death and donation and what it made her believe about the big question at hand, which was this: 'Should it be easier to harvest organs for transplant?'

Sue didn't like that word – 'harvest'. Nor did a couple of the doctors on the panel either, it turned out as they chatted before the show in the staffroom of the school where the debate was being held. There was coffee and pastries and apples and bananas in a bowl with oranges too, although she wondered who on earth was going to eat one of those messy things before going on live television. Sue had chosen a black and white print dress and a matching gold necklace and earrings. She had been to have her hair done for this, as a way of finding the confidence.

The host, Nicky Campbell, was tall and formidable in a black suit and an open-necked white shirt and he was circulating the room, giving everybody a few minutes before the show. Sue thought he was trying to get the measure of them all. A researcher said it was time to go through, so she took a last swig of water, breathed deeply and followed. She was amused to see that beyond the pool of studio lighting and the stage dressing it was just a big old draughty school hall.

'Don't look at the monitors while we're on air, or you'll look daft,' the presenter told them all as a technician attached a microphone to her collar. An imam was sitting next to her, jammed up against her shoulder, and he gave her a nice smile. Professor Dawkins was smiling to himself as the presenter launched into his introduction and Sue felt a surge of nerves. 'Doctors are now asking whether donors can be kept on ventilation to preserve their organs for longer,' said Nicky Campbell and she thought about the long night and day that Martin had been lying there, pink and warm but dead already, waiting for his dad to come and say goodbye and for the surgical teams to be ready. She was grateful for the extra time with him, but to have gone on for another day would have been torture.

'He's a hero for what he's done for others,' said the presenter, now talking about Martin and looking straight down at her. People applauded. This was her cue. Her mouth was dry and her voice was shaky but she did manage to get the words out: 'You've got a very short space of time to make a decision you will have to live with for the rest of your life. Whether you agree to it or not, whether you say yes or no, it is important not to regret that.'

The doctors had been sensitive and supportive and made it feel like a positive decision, she said, but it was still awful to have to think about organ donation when you had just been told your son was brain dead. There should be a campaign to make people more informed in advance. 'People need to talk about it around the dinner table when there is no emergency, before they are sat in ICU with a member of their family who is dying.'

Everyone clapped again, including Professor Dawkins, who declared: 'Well said indeed. These are very, very difficult matters.' The grey-haired scientist pulled out a donor card and waved it in the air. 'The doctors' and the patients' lives would be made a lot easier if everybody carried one of these!' That was very popular and drew more applause, as he had known it would. Then the presenter moved along to an intensive care consultant that Sue had met before, who talked about how collecting the organs and delivering them to the patients straight away was one of the most complicated processes performed anywhere in the National Health Service. 'It takes anything up to twenty-four hours to organise multiple surgical teams from around the country to come to the hospital, while recipients are getting phone calls telling them to go to their hospitals now. The family of a dying person is there the whole time. Twenty-four hours is an eternity for those people.'

The next speaker was a young woman called Amy, who was waiting for a double lung transplant. There was a plastic tube in her nose to help her breathe and she looked very pale, but Amy was forceful. Four out of ten potential donors had their will denied by their families, she said, because the living didn't respect the wishes of the dead or just couldn't go through with it. Amy wanted a new system that assumed everyone was willing to give up their organs unless they opted out. She said she felt bad waiting for someone to die, but Sue wasn't having that.

'You're not waiting for someone to die, Amy,' she said urgently, leaning forward, trying to look her in the eye. 'You're waiting for someone who is going to die anyway, and for their family to say "yes".'

Her heart was beating fast now, but the discussion moved on. The imam next to her was waving his hands in her space, saying he would never carry a donor card.

'There should be a card that says "Don't take my organs after my death!"'

Sue bristled at that, what was he on about?

'Not every Muslim knows that in the holy book, the Qur'an, it says that my hand, my feet, my ear, my vision, my skin will record every deed I do in this life, good or bad. On the Day of Judgement, my account will be put by my organs.'

She had never heard that before, but now another Muslim was contradicting him. He was younger, with kind eyes, and he had a different reading of the Qur'an. 'That's too simplistic. The organs don't have to be near you to testify. God needs to see your spiritual heart, not your actual heart. As a Muslim, I believe I have been put here to do good.'

He would donate his organs and he would certainly want them to be available if he or his family fell ill. There was a Christian too, who agreed. 'I see human beings as gifts to each other and that's why we are here. We exist in a community, we have obligations to each other.' A sweaty guy on the end of the row, dressed all in black, was there for a different debate on the same show but was trying to say he had been persuaded to think about carrying a donor card. He stumbled over his words and they ran out of time.

Sue was relieved it was all over, although she was concerned that she had not done very well and she said so to the guy in black as they were led back to the green room to pick up their stuff, before taxis took them home. He tried to be reassuring – I know that because he was me. This is where I step into the story I have been telling up until now, as this was the day I met Sue and began to hear about Martin.

I had always been squeamish about the idea of anything – heart, lungs, liver, kidneys or corneas, whatever – being taken from my body after death. It stirred up feelings I didn't understand, but nobody had ever forced me to confront them. Listening to Sue, I was challenged to start thinking it all through rather than avoiding the issue, and she asked a question of her own that cut right through the core of it all.

'If your child was dying and the only thing that could save them was an organ from someone else, would you want them to have it?'

'Yes, of course,' I said, being honest.

'Then how can you deny that to someone else after you've gone?'

My personal feelings about organ donation began to change at that moment. And although neither of us knew it at the time, Sue's appearance on television that morning was about to change her own life too, dramatically.

THIRTY-ONE

LINDA

'What the hell?' Linda woke up on the Sunday morning to the sound of her mobile ringing on the bedside table and when she groped for the phone and found it she saw ten missed calls from her mum. Something must be wrong. Everyone in the house was asleep, so she kept her voice down – and it was always croaky enough anyway first thing in the morning – when she called back.

'Mum, what is it?'

'Linda, I am deadly serious, hen. I think I have just seen Marc's donor's mum on the television. I am not joking, something drew me to this woman.'

'What do you mean?'

'I've just got this feeling. You better switch it on, hen, right now.'

So Linda turned on the television and saw Sue on *The Big Questions* talking about Martin. The caption under her name mentioned the Donor Family Network charity, which got Linda thinking: 'Right, there's my lead. I'll find them and I can find her.' And she did.

Nigel was actually the first to get a message. 'I had a friend request from a Linda McCay on Facebook, but then I get quite a few because of the charity. Sue was not on Facebook at that time. I didn't really appreciate who the person was but I accepted it and thought, "Whatever". Then she posted something. I read the post and the penny dropped. I thought, "I know who you are. You're Marc's mum."'

The post was actually a link to an article I had written about Sue and Andrew, who had got Martin's liver. Sue was a bit shocked to see it there. 'I looked on Linda's Facebook timeline and the first thing I saw was a picture of Martin. She had used the picture from the article and said, "Follow this link to read the story of Marc's donor." It was scary. You know these things are out there in the public domain but it is quite alarming when you go onto someone else's timeline and see the face of your child.'

The two mothers began to email each other, sending long messages about their families and giving their own accounts of what happened in August 2003.

They compared dates and had a lot to talk about, although having been so keen to get in touch, Linda now found herself holding back, emotionally.

'For a long time I felt guilty, and when we started corresponding I didn't tell her how I felt. I had lived for years with that guilt, because the year to the day after Martin had collapsed – as I now knew – my first grandson had been born. Leasa's son Robert was like a gift from God to me, but I felt, "How can I tell that woman who has lost her son that I have still got my four sons and now I have got a grandson as well?" I was still crying for her and I was not very good at holding it together. So I had to be careful what I said to her, I didn't want to cause her any more pain.'

The feelings were raw. They were three hundred miles apart and the moment never seemed right so the Burtons and the McCays did not meet ... until Lynne Holt intervened, unexpectedly. This busy, bustling organiser who led a nursing team at the Freeman also worked with a charity called Transplant Sport and she had an offer to make. A company in Canada called the Rocky Mountaineer was inviting the families of donors and those who had received organs to ride together on what it called a Train for Heroes. They would be flown out to Canada and given hotel rooms, great food and drink and a two-day ride on a luxuri-ous train with a glass roof so that everything was on view as they passed through some of the most spectacular scenery on earth, from Vancouver to a place called Lake Louise, deep in the Rockies. This would help raise awareness of Transplant Sport and just be a great thing to do. On top of that, if the Burtons agreed to go then the company would make the same offer to the McCays. 'I had never been involved with a situation like this before,' says Lynne Holt. 'As a mother myself, I felt for Sue and for Linda. I was emotionally involved with this now. The donor families say they are not brave, because they made the only decision they could make and it comforts them knowing that good comes out of their loss, but they are brave really. So it was wonderful to be able to say thank you and to give them the experience of a lifetime.'

As long as both families agreed to the trip, they were going to meet at last.

THIRTY-TWO

MARC & SUE

'Why don't you take a stethoscope? You could listen to his heart.'

Sue laughed at the suggestion from one of the secretaries at work. She was not going to ask a boy she had just met to lift up his shirt so she could press a cold metal instrument against his bare chest, thank you very much. That would be too embarrassing and more than a bit weird. Her head was already swirling. What would it be like to hear her son's heart beating away inside another boy, who was the same age as Martin and living the life he had been denied? She almost couldn't bear to think about that. On the other hand, she couldn't stop thinking about him either. 'I did wonder how I was going to cope. At the back of my mind, I did wish Martin still had that heart. Of course I did. I wouldn't be a mother if I didn't feel like that.'

Sue would have been nervous if they had just been going for coffee somewhere low-key, but this was turning into a big production. They weren't meeting at a Costa in a service station halfway between her house and his. Oh no, that was too simple. They were going all the way to Canada, of all places. The McCays had accepted the same invitation and travelled separately, staying in a different hotel on the first night. But now they were in Canada and it was time for them to meet.

'Marc's inside. Are you ready for this?'

The question came from the boss of the *Rocky Mountaineer*, who was giving the adventure of a lifetime. The long blue-and-gold train had a glass dome roof that would allow them to see some of the most spectacular scenery in the world. There might be eagles soaring overhead, fish leaping in wide lakes and bears in the deep forests and there would definitely be breathtaking mountains with high, snow-capped peaks to watch over them, mirrored in the wide lakes. All of that was very nice, but it wasn't what Sue had come for. It wasn't what got her really excited: that was the prospect of meeting Linda and Marc, who were waiting inside the vast, airport-style terminal at the train station. The train would not be leaving until the next day so the check-in desks were empty and there was nobody else about, it was just going to be the Burtons and the McCays, together for the first time. Sue knew Marc and Linda from photographs, so she instantly recognised the slight, pale boy with the sandy hair and his mother beside him, wringing her hands, smiling nervously.

'We could see them in the distance, through the glass doors. They stood up when they saw us. I could sense Nigel falling back slightly behind me as we went in and I could see that Linda was doing exactly the same with Marc, so I thought, "Okay, mate, it's you and me …"'

Her first instinct was to open her arms and run over, but Sue had thought long and hard about this. 'What do you do? This poor young man might not want some middle-aged woman throwing herself at him, he might not like that – I knew my eldest would hate it – so I was prepared to be quite calm.'

The station hall was huge, with a high ceiling and light flooding in through tall windows. Sue forced herself to hold back, walk steadily across the polished floor towards him and let Marc take the lead. 'I was determined not to be over-the-top, but as we got nearer he just ran for me and slung himself at me and hugged me and I was like, "That's fine, mate. I can do hugs! I can do hugs, I just wasn't sure you'd want to." And he hugged me and he cried.'

That was relief surging through him, said Marc afterwards. 'I'd been getting more and more nervous about what I would say then Sue arrived and I felt the tears coming, so all I could do was shoot towards her. I didn't know what else to do but say thanks and cuddle her and that was it.'

Sue hugged him back, not knowing how to feel.

'I remember saying to him, "Can I go and give your mum a hug now?"'

The two mothers embraced for a long time, each feeling instantly as if they had found someone who understood some of what they had been through. They talked all afternoon, then they talked all night at a dinner for the families and they were still talking when the *Rocky Mountaineer* set off the next day. 'Linda and I had so much to talk about on the train over the next few days that by the time we got to Lake Louise we knew exactly what had happened to each other and our families. We knew the whole story.'

Marc was happy to let them get on with it. The shy lad from Renfrewshire watched out of the window as the train sped through valleys, over dizzyingly high bridges and by the sides of great lakes. When Marc felt like chatting he turned to Nigel, who kept it light. 'We just talked about football, like guys do.'

Sue missed a lot of the scenery, she was so engrossed in conversation with Linda and some of the forty or so other passengers on their part of the train who had their own experiences of organ donation. They were from Britain, Australia and the United States as well as Canada, although there was only one other case of a donor family and recipient being brought together. 'We were on a high because of what we were doing. I think it's the simple fact that when you've been through something so big and emotional, you actually thrive on talking about it, even though that sounds terribly exhausting. There was lot of partying ...'

A handsome young waiter caught the attention of some of the women, who got him to make cocktails for them, says Sue. 'We'd be sitting there drinking Zac's special cocktail, "Zac's Surprise", and making a lot of noise. There was a lot of laughter. It's that camaraderie of sharing your story, and speaking to someone who's been through something similar, that is actually quite strengthening. To actually know that someone understands.'

Sometimes, though, she went off on her own to the open platform at the back of the train, for a bit of quiet. 'My tears were clearly for my loss, clearly for Martin, who would have been the same age as Marc. I don't think I could have met Marc any sooner, without really wanting it to have been Martin who was alive instead.'

Linda was full of gratitude, saying she knew how lucky Marc was. 'We could so easily have been in the same position as you.'

Sue kept looking over at Marc, thinking about how well he seemed. Thinking about how Martin would have been at that age. 'I did struggle with that at first but it was all right in the end, very different from what I had feared. Linda was lovely and it was amazing to see the person who had benefitted from our decision all those years ago. I was glad Marc was doing so well.'

They met by the side of Lake Louise on their last day together: fellow passengers who had lost a father, mother, sister, brother, son or daughter and those who had been saved by a stranger's heart, lungs or other organs. Each of them was asked to pick up a smooth pebble from a wicker basket, turn it over in their hands and think of somebody who was missed. Some kissed their stone before they threw it out over the water, watching the splash and the ripples. Every person there knew very well how the splash of the end of one life can ripple out to touch the lives of many others.

When the short ceremony was over, the Burtons and the McCays went walking together by the strikingly blue lake. The water was still again now, reflecting the v-shape of the sky between snowy mountains that looked too perfect to be real. Marc was nervous once more, knowing there was something he wanted to do for Sue. They were getting towards their last moments together, before they had to go their separate ways and go home. It took him a while to pluck up the courage, but when they stopped for a photograph, the four of them arm-in-arm, he seized the moment. Sue was taken by surprise. 'Marc suddenly just took my hand and put it on his heart. He was only wearing a thin T-shirt, while I was in a heavy coat. Obviously the heart keeps him warm!' she says, hesitating over the memory even now. It was so quick, but it meant so much to her. 'He put my hand on his heart. The skin was thin because of all the wounds he had there from the operations and I could really feel the heart beating. That was a very special moment.'

Then it was gone. Somebody spoke, it was time to go and pack. The moment slipped by, all too brief and never to be repeated. Or so they thought at the time ...

THIRTY-THREE

MARC

Marc is about to open the door. He should have died. By the old standards, he was dead on the operating table: his heart did not just stop beating, it was cut out and thrown away. Yet here he is, more than a dozen years later, in the doorway of his apartment on a cold, grey day. 'You better come in,' he says, with a handshake so shy it's apologetic. 'You found us okay? You need a car to stay here, public transport's not too good.' He lives in Lochwinnoch, a small village in lovely countryside twenty miles to the west of Glasgow, where the McCay children all grew up. 'It's in the middle of nowhere and when the two lochs join up in the floods we can't get out, but I love it.'

His voice is flutey, he's clearly anxious. 'I haven't got the words,' he says, but that's fair enough. You can't expect a young man of twenty-eight to have the language to describe a miracle perfectly just because it's happening in his chest eighty times a minute, four thousand eight hundred beats an hour. 'I've never talked to anyone about this properly before.' This is the first time we have met, so why has he agreed to talk now? 'Sue said you were okay. That's good enough for me.'

His eyes are a clear, striking green. His mother was right: Marc is a good-looking guy. All the operations and pills have reduced his strength, slimmed him right down and at the same time made his face a little puffed and blotchy, but despite all of that, he remains handsome. He's made an effort to look good today, with his box-fresh blue sneakers, crisp jeans and a long-sleeved T-shirt with a vintage skyline of Manhattan and the words Twisted Soul. That's a label, not the state of his being. Marc is cheerful and friendly, despite his nerves. The rented apartment is simply furnished, with plain walls and not much furniture apart from a black sofa and a matching armchair and a big television screen with games console underneath. He shares the place with a friend, who is out just now. They play a lot of combat games, pretending to be battle-hardened, super-fit troops. He likes online poker to get through all the restless nights when his body groans and complains and keeps him awake.

He's happy enough, he says. 'Life is good. I have a great time with my mates and my family. All these years when I shouldn't have been here, there have been some great laughs. I'm like Rangers, my football club: on the up again after not doing so good for a while.'

So we start to talk about what happened to him. I know more than he does about where his heart came from and the bravery, compassion and love that came with it, but I want to hear things from his point of view. 'I never had anything wrong with me in my life before I got sick. Nothing. I never even knew what sick was, to be honest. I was at that age where you didn't think of stuff like that – you just wanted to go with your life and play sport and be the best at everything.'

On the day his mum rushed him to hospital in August 2003, the stomach pains overtook him faster than the fear. 'I was just taking paracetamol, thinking, "It'll go away in the morning." My mum said, "You need to go the doctors." I was in agony. I was being sick. We couldn't understand what was wrong at all.'

He was just unlucky, I say. Marc smiles and shakes his head. 'No, I was lucky. The doctor told me, "You better start doing the lottery. Fifteen out of forty million people a year get this virus, so that's really bad luck, but only four of those survive. So if you make it, you're really lucky.'"

Maybe he should buy a lottery ticket?

'I don't want to use up all my luck, I might need it.'

He doesn't recall much of his time unconscious in hospital, for obvious reasons, but Marc does remember hearing his mum crying – or greeting, to use the Scots word. 'I heard her greeting, non-stop. I can remember that, but I don't know how. It was weird to just wake up round all these English people. It was a bit crazy, all these accents, a different country. I had a big ventilator down my throat, I couldn't even ask any questions. I was lying flat. I couldn't move, I couldn't speak. Nobody I knew was near me.' That's when he had the hallucinations. 'I woke up and a woman was injecting stuff in me. I was scared she was trying to kill me.'

Even when he began to come round properly, it was a while before he recognised that his mum and dad were in the room. 'They had to explain to me what had happened and at the same time I was only fifteen, I was thinking, "What the hell is a heart transplant?" I didn't know. Then I was just thinking, "Okay, cool, can you let me out? Can I go home?" It was the weirdest thing in the world ever.'

They told Marc how close he had been to death. 'I must've been as close as you can get, I reckon. My heart was enlarged three times bigger than it was meant to be and that was crushing all my organs inside my body. Getting the heart transplant, having my heart taken out, I must have pretty much died.'

Does he know what had happened to his old heart? 'I never asked.'

Move on, look to the future, that is his way. The flabby, swollen heart was probably incinerated at the hospital mortuary. The most highly regarded part of his body was destroyed long before his actual death. Strange to think of the ashes going up a chimney to scatter in the air above Newcastle, a long way from his home, like a human sacrifice to some distant god. Losing your heart was the definition of death for eight thousand years, until medical science intervened and people like Marc became living, breathing marvels. According to the traditional understanding of several faiths, his soul should have left his body when his original heart stopped beating. Yet here he is, still Marc. His accent has not mysteriously changed to English. He hasn't started supporting West Ham like Martin. He hasn't developed any of his donor's lovely puppy dog enthusiasm, an idea that amuses him. 'I am a really laid-back person, so I kind of just get on with it. I try to stay positive. My mum says she is glad it happened to me and not one of the other brothers as they aren't as laid-back as me. One of them is scared of needles, he can't be in hospital. He got paranoid after what happened to me and got chest pains as well so he was really freaking out, but it turned out to be anxiety. All my family got tested and everyone else's hearts are fine.'

The recovery process was just like a footballer working hard to return to fitness; that's how he tried to think of it he says, only it was a bit more extreme. 'I couldn't even walk or anything. I had to learn again. All the muscles inside my legs had disappeared so I had to build them back up: go in a swimming pool and walk length to length. I got out of breath so easily, but other than that, everything went fine. I was worried about taking all the pills, thinking, "I'm never going to get used to this." But it got easier as the days went by.'

Now, let's ask the question that so very few people in history can answer. What is it like to have some-body else's heart inside your body? 'I try not to think about it.' He gives a weak little smile and looks away, but I don't believe him. Not one bit. Sue briefly felt the scars and the damaged, thin skin on his chest and was shocked at how easy it was to feel his heart under-neath, so come on, surely he puts his own hand there sometimes and wonders at it all? 'I do that, aye. If I'm lying in my bed at night on my own I can feel it beat-ing, in a way I don't think other people can. I've asked them. They just let their hearts get on with it, they never know what's going on, like I was before all this. Can you feel yours?'

'No, I can't,' I say. I try, while I'm sitting here with him, but there's nothing.

'Okay, well, most of the time there's nothing for most people, right? But I can feel it all the time. When I lie awake, I feel it strong. I know when it mistimes a beat. Sometimes it feels like it's popping out of my chest. It's insane to think that this is in me now when it was in Martin before.'

He's got his hand on his heart now, flat against it. Does it feel like part of his own body or something else, something extra? 'Something else. Definitely. I mean, I couldn't live without it and it's part of me but it's like they opened a door and put the heart in and it's locked in there, helping me out.'

All this makes his head spin. 'It is a lot to cope with. You get some patients who think about the heart transplant and the operation all the time and it just puts stress and worry into their head thinking something's going to go wrong and they'll need another one. I think people worry too much instead of just getting on with it and enjoying the heart they've got. I try and forget about it. I don't mean forget about Martin and his family, of course not. I just mean try to get on with your normal life.'

Would that have been easier if the two mothers had never made contact and he had never found out so much about his donor? 'Aye, I think so. But I don't mind. I'm glad for them.' What then did he think or feel when he first saw a photograph of Martin? 'It was weird, he reminded me of myself when I was fifteen. We were a bit similar, with the blond hair and I was stocky like him at that age. He was into his football like me, like any young boy. We were alike. It was kind of crazy.'

Does he talk to his heart? He laughs, as if that is a crazy idea, but I tell him that Andrew Seery sometimes talks to his liver and calls it Martin. 'I don't know how to react to that,' says Marc, looking embarrassed. Something is nagging at him, I can see that, but he changes the subject for now. We talk about religion, which is so much part of the place where he lives and grew up. Rangers versus Celtic, blue versus green, Protestant versus Catholic, all those old feelings that his great-grandparents defied when they fell in love but that still burst into life sometimes in punch-ups and bar brawls or worse. 'I had all that. I went to Sunday school when I was a kid but I never really thought about it and what happens next – you know, if there's a heaven and that – until I had my dream.' That was when he met his father, his grandfather and old John McCay, who was a stranger to him at the time.

'When I asked about him they told me he died twenty-two years before. That was really weird, it did freak me out, because I know I had never seen him before in my life but when I saw a photo it was the same person. So deep down now, I do kind of think there is something there after we die. Hopefully, aye.' Not many of us get so close to finding out as he did. 'Aye, exactly. The dream made me think there's something out there. I feel as though I've been there. That's what makes me think something else the way I do, which is really personal but I do believe it.' He looks away again, shy. What does he mean, what is it that he believes? 'That Martin is here with me too. Really. All the time.'

Now that he knows I'm not going to laugh at him or call him daft, Marc has something to confess. 'I do talk to Martin. Rather than to the heart, do you know what I mean? As though he's still around. If I have a funny day, I would have a wee talk to Martin and I just say stuff to him.'

What sort of stuff?

'Make me better, please. Make my health good.'

That's what his mum does too. They wouldn't put it like this, but Martin has become like their own personal saint, the person in heaven they can ask to put in a good word with the boss.

'I've always been fine, so hopefully somebody's there watching, keeping us alright. If I'm feeling ill, I just say, "Let's get through this. Let's do this." It sounds funny, but aye, I have. It's both ways. I've got his heart so I feel as if Martin must be there, looking down on me, going, "Make sure my heart's all right."'

Without realising it, Marc still has his hand on his heart.

'I don't understand it, but I do feel like he's looking out for me, for real.'

Football is his great love, the thing in life that gives him more joy than anything else. For a while, when he was strong enough after the transplant, he did incredibly well at the game again. 'I wasn't as fit as I wanted to be but I was just happy to be playing. A couple of the boys used to say I was one of the best players ever to play with the village team – and that was with the new heart, which was good to hear.' So he was back in the game and it was wonderful, until the day he collapsed. That was in 2009 and Marc ended up back in hospital: this time a specialist heart failure unit at the Golden Jubilee National Hospital near Glasgow. His arteries had narrowed, which often happens to heart transplant patients, and so again the flow of his blood was being slowed down and oxygen was not getting to his system in the way it should. The doctors sent another one of those long, thin, flexible tubes up an artery into the heart and they inflated a little balloon to widen the artery then fitted a tiny mesh stent to keep it like that. Slowly, Marc was able to recover.

Now he is playing with his brothers on the five-a-side pitch at Lochwinnoch again every week, hoping to get back to the full-size game. 'I still have a good touch, a good shot, a good pass, but I can't do too much running. The whole team knows I have had a heart transplant, so they try to cover me and not let me do too much.' He can still handle the rough stuff, though. 'They know I can take a tackle. The only thing is, every time I get a kick I get covered in bruises, because of the blood thinners. But that's fine, I can handle a wee kick every now and again.'

There's just one thing holding him back. 'I am getting bad stomach problems and they can't figure out what is. The doctors said this problem will just pass and some days I am fine, but some days I get really bad cramp in my belly.'

His pills for the day are lined up in a row on the coffee table, red and yellow and blue. 'There's a couple of immune suppressant drugs. There's the one to stop my body rejecting the heart and a couple of blood thinners. My heart rate can go too high, so there's beta blockers to keep it at a nice rate. There are pills to help my arteries, I think. Twelve different kinds of pills in the morning and seven before bed. It is a nightmare trying to remember to take them all, but if it's going to keep me alive then I don't mind.'

I ask if he is able to work and he says it has been frustrating. 'As soon as I started kicking a ball again I started working. I had an apprenticeship, a landscape gardening job, so I was doing quite well with that but then I ended getting paid off.'

His next job was in a call centre. 'It was quite stressful, phoning people up and trying to sell them broadband. I gave that up, it wasn't good for my heart. This last year I have kind of been on hold because of my stomach. I would love to be out there making money of course, now is the only time I have not had a car. I'll try and get a job when my belly's better, but sometimes it's a nightmare, I just can't do anything.'

He's not a shirker, by any means. Marc wants to be useful, so he has been helping a mate out at the sports centre, painting the walls. 'I only have to stand with a brush and paint, it's not like I have to walk or anything. I would do anything to get a proper job and start working again, just these stomach pains are annoying. I shouldn't complain though. My heart is working really well. I've never had any rejection, touch wood.'

He'd rather talk about the good stuff than dwell on his problems. 'See, I was all but dead. I've had all these years I wouldn't have had if it wasn't for Martin and

I'm gonna have more so I just want to get on and be happy, enjoy myself, make the most of it. For him as much as me.'

He's not lonely, you couldn't say that. Marc lives with his friend, and his brothers and sister, Mum and Dad and nephews and nieces are all nearby. Most of the mates he has had since he was a small boy still live in this village or the surrounding towns – there is a gang of them and they go out together all the time, to the pub or the match or to a casino. 'The house always wins, you know that? But I don't always lose!'

I'm wondering about his love life, though. Marc is at an age when some lads start thinking about settling down and having kids. His dad had four by this age. Norrie has already told me a little bit of the story. 'Marc had a few women friends, you know, even after what happened to him. He always had a way about him. Then this lassie came along and it was serious. They were good for each other. She was a nurse, although not one that was treating him, and her father was a doctor.'

They were very close and into each other and went about life in their own way to match her shift work and his condition. Norrie saw a romantic side in Marc that clearly didn't come from him. 'I couldn't get my head around the two of them sometimes. They'd be making soup at three in the morning. They were very lovey-dovey, you know?'

When I ask Marc about this, his pale cheeks actually acquire a soft pink blush. 'Well, I had a girlfriend for about four years but that stopped a good year or two ago.'

Marc does not want to talk about it, except to say that he loved her very much and always will. He hopes to have children one day, but he's still young and for the time being Marc has given up on looking for another girlfriend. 'Since then I just can't be bothered anymore. I do my own thing.' Being Marc, he tries to make light of it all. 'See, when I had a girlfriend I didn't look after my health, because I was too worried about her and trying to look after her. I'd rather be single and look after myself and worry about my own health.' The feelings are still very raw, clearly. Confused, too. He's not over that relationship, the love endures, but it is some kind of relief not to have to fret about someone else. Marc wants a normal life, but he is a sensitive guy who doesn't want to hurt anyone. He has seen the people he loves suffer because of his illness and he is wary of putting somebody new through all of that.

On the other hand, he knows he needs help sometimes, but he doesn't want to be smothered. Marc loves his mum with all his being, but he doesn't want the same thing from a girlfriend. So it's tricky, finding the right person, and for now he is not looking. 'I do want to be with someone and maybe have kids, but not yet. I've got time, hopefully. I need to be my own man a little bit now, you know?'

I've spoken to his little brother Daryl, who says Marc is still a bit of a charmer with the opposite sex, even if he's not after anyone just now. 'Girls like that easy-ozeyness about him, they can just relax. He's like that with the wains, too.' That's the Scots word for children, and Marc is great with them. He is particularly close to Leasa's son Robert, his nephew, who comes round to see him nearly every day. They play a lot of games on the console, says Daryl. 'Marc never really got the chance to grow up properly because of what happened. He's always had that bit of daftness and immaturity about him, which is great.'

Daryl is now in his early twenties, and the youngest son has been the first member of the family to go to university. He has a good job helping to design ships, lives with a partner and has a couple of young children, who love their Uncle Marc. In some ways he has overtaken his brother in life, although he would never say so. They see a lot of each other, but they keep things light. 'He'd be like, "Did you watch the football last night? How are the wains getting on?" Then maybe we'd give each other a wee slagging or two, as brothers do.' Daryl is just glad to have Marc around to hang out with. 'We need to cherish that, rather than think about the negatives. Nigel and Sue would have loved to have had these extra years with Martin. We've had some brilliant times together.'

Marc agrees, totally. 'We were talking about being lucky but I do feel as if I have won the lottery. There are still a lot of struggles but that's still better than the alternative, you know? I've had all this life I wouldn't have had. What I went through has probably made me a better person too. I was kind of the spoiled one for the first few years after I got the transplant, but I do think it's made us a lot closer.'

From what I have seen of the McCays, that's true. This is a close, loving family and they are all rooting for Marc. Today, they all know he's a bit nervous. When we finish talking, he is going to meet Sue again for the first time since the *Rocky Mountaineer*.

'When I'm with her, I don't really know what to say. I just freeze. I would rather write it down on a card and tell her what I think that way, because I'm not really good at talking. I don't really know what you're meant to say. How are you meant to thank someone for giving you a heart? It's the biggest gift anybody could ever give anybody. If I did win the actual lottery I'd give it all to them. That's how I feel. They've kept me alive.'

'Why not say that, then?'

Marc laughs.

'No matter how many times you say thanks, it's still not ever going to be enough.'

THIRTY-FOUR

SUE & LINDA

Here come the mums. We're outside the country hotel where Linda works now and the weather is foul. It's a cold, dark, wet and windy day but the warmth between these two is obvious as soon as they meet. Sue, the quiet Englishwoman, opens her arms to Linda and the passionate, fiery Scot engulfs her in a hug. How can they love each other like this, against all the odds? How can a mother who has lost her son become mates with the mother of the boy who has his heart? It's not allowed and it never happens – and yet in this case it has and here they are, very close friends reunited. They are so very different, even in the way they speak. Sue is naturally cautious and nibbles at her words, Linda rolls them around her mouth like they're really tasty, but the two of them are chatting away within moments. They should be chalk and cheese, but they somehow go together like cheese and wine.

'I think it's a friendship but it's also a special bond, something that you would never expect to have under normal circumstances,' says Sue, who is going to meet Marc again shortly but wants to spend some time with his mum first. Their closeness began as soon as they met on the *Rocky Mountaineer*, she says. They talked and talked and kept the conversation going afterwards on Facebook. 'I feel like she understands some of what I have been through and I am the same with her.'

We go inside the lodge to get out of the rain and it's comfortable, cosy.

'The two of us have a very special bond. I do believe we were on the same journey in life,' says Linda. 'We can match our stories up, she can tell me where she was on the same day.'

On that awful Tuesday night in August 2003, Linda was on her way down to Newcastle, desperately praying for a miracle for her dying son, when Sue was just home from the swimming pool, sitting on the sofa at home in Grantham with her happy, healthy boy, blissfully unaware of what was about to happen.

Then when Martin was suddenly and cruelly snatched away from her by a brain bleed and the doctors in Nottingham told her on the Wednesday that there was no chance at all of him surviving, Linda was pacing the corridors of the Freeman Hospital three hundred miles away, hoping for a new heart to become available somewhere, from someone. And of course it did, at a terrible cost.

On the Thursday night, they both said goodbye to their sons. Linda knew Marc was going for an operation that could save him or kill him. Sue knew she had lost Martin forever. 'I am jealous of her for having her son alive, of course I am, that is only natural. I would not be a mother otherwise. But I also know that we both believed we were losing our child that night. Linda was heading towards that, she was expecting Marc not to live. Even when the heart became available, there was no way of knowing if Marc would make it. I find it incredible that she actually had it in her, at that time, to think of us.'

When Linda saw the heart arrive at the Freeman she felt a great surge of compassion for the family of the boy who had died, whoever and wherever they might have been. But now Sue says she has realised for the first time that she actually thought of Linda too, without knowing her. 'There was nothing I could do for Martin any more but when I was asked about organ donation I remember distinctly thinking, "If I can save another mother from going through this then that is what I need to do." When we found out about Marc a day later, it all fell into place. I thought, "Well, there is another mother out there, she is my age, her son is the same as Martin, it all makes sense, this is right."'

They're drinking tea from the hotel mugs. Sue is on the sofa with her legs crossed, still a little anxious for the right words. She fiddles with the heavy green beads of her necklace, hanging over a purple top. Linda is on the other side of the room in black boots and jeans and a long, cream dress top with lace edges. Her straight, blonde hair frames her face as she speaks, quickly, eager to let her feelings spill out. 'I felt so guilty when I first got in touch with Sue through emails and Facebook, but she was saying to me, "Linda, don't feel guilty." I remember saying to my daughter, "It's as if she knows me." But then she is a mum and we have walked the same path.'

Linda does not think she could have coped with the grief as well as Sue. 'I would have been in a corner somewhere, honestly. I know my own self, my own mind, and it would be too much. My children are my life.' She glances across as if to check it is okay to say this and is answered with a sympathetic smile. 'Even as an adult, I am still running about, caring for them. No matter what their age, you're always a mother.'

Those words bring Sue close to tears. 'You have no choice. You have to get through. You learn to live with yourself and embrace this new life. There is almost an element of peace, despite the fact that I miss Martin every day and I still grieve for him every day. I think it is important not to sit in a corner and wallow in the grief but to say, "This is not me, my grief does not define me."'

She twists a paper hankie with her fingers. Becoming a grandmother has helped Sue heal. 'I did wonder how would I feel when my son and his wife had children, because how can you ever give love to that depth when you've lost someone? You're actually frightened to ever let yourself love again, because something awful might happen. I used to fear that. But the day the first grandchild was born, that just disappeared. When you spend time with young children you can't help but just focus entirely on them because that's what they need. They're in your face.'

Hearing her talk like this, in such an open and emotional way, gives Linda the confidence to share something that has been on her mind. 'I remember when Marc was getting better and he was even able to play football again after a few years and he scored his first goal. I looked up to the heavens and said, "Thank you, God." Then I was like, "Oh Martin, I wish your mum and dad could see that." That goal was for both him and Martin.'

Sue looks a little taken aback by the full force of Linda's emotion, but she answers anyway. 'It's actually really important to know things like that. It helps families like us understand that the decision we made in the time of our own trauma was the right one.'

Linda has gone quiet. What is she thinking? 'No, you're all right,' she says, dismissively. They chat for a while about the hotel and what Linda does there as a housekeeper and what their children are up to. My friend Jonathan is with us, because I've already started to write about this and he is a producer who wants to help them tell their story on the radio. The strong thoughts and feelings inside Linda never stay hidden for long, and so they come spilling out now. 'I'm sitting here thinking Marc has got that heart inside him. That heart grew inside Sue for nine months. That was Nigel's and Sue's baby that they made. Now Marc has got part of him, that's just the way I feel. They gave my son life. Now Marc has got two mums.'

She's looking over here, avoiding eye contact with Sue. Linda gives a little nervous chuckle, as if regretting what she just said, but she can't back down now. 'If the roles were reversed, as a mum, that is how I would feel. If we were sitting here right now and that was Martin coming in the door and Marc was gone, I think I would feel, "That heart grew inside me for nine months." You know?'

Sue nods. She is not fazed. Perhaps she has heard it before. Perhaps the same thought has occurred to her.

But Linda feels uneasy and makes a joke of it. 'I just mean metaphorically speaking, I don't mean full, hands-on Sue is his other mum. God help him, he's got enough with me!'

They both laugh. Sue stands up and reaches out for Linda again and they meet each other halfway across the room and hug. There are tears. But now Marc is coming and Sue needs to compose herself. We were talking about this in the car on the way up, so I know what a big deal it is going to be. There is unfinished business between them. That moment by Lake Louise in Canada when he took her hand and put it on his chest so she could feel his heart was wonderful, but it was also sudden, unsettling and over far too soon.

THIRTY-FIVE

MARC & SUE

N ow here it is. The moment. A happy ending of
sorts in this story of horrors, trials and wonders.
They have not seen each other since Canada, but
Marc and Sue are together at last on a sofa in the
lodge at the hotel in the Scottish countryside where
his mum works as a housekeeper. The night has
come but the lamps in here cast a golden glow. This
is the first time they have sat down properly to talk
about everything that happened and Sue knows what
she wants to say. It sounds like a prepared speech,
because she has rehearsed this in her mind many
times. 'I don't want you to feel guilty because Martin
died and you lived. Martin was going to die anyway.
We agreed to donate his organs when he died and we
are thrilled to know that lives have been saved
because of him.'

Marc looks uneasy, unsure how to respond. He is grateful, of course, for everything that has happened, but struggles for a way to express that. He still has health problems, a transplant can't solve them all, but he feels fitter than he has for years. All this would have been too much to hope or pray for a dozen years ago when his mum was pacing the hospital corridors pleading with God to take her life in return for his, as she often reminded him. Marc is a bit overwhelmed by Sue's presence when he sees her again, as he had said he would be when we met earlier. 'How are you supposed to thank somebody for giving you a heart? It's the biggest gift anyone could give, and there's no way to say thanks.'

Perhaps there is a way, though. Actions might speak louder than words. Would he allow her to place her hand on his chest again?

'You're getting me embarrassed now,' he says bashfully, as if he wants to refuse. But he can see Sue wants to do it. The answer has to be yes.

'I'm getting upset now,' she says with a sniff, but shuffles up closer to him.

Slowly, awkwardly, assuming that it's all right, she reaches across him, as if to lay hands in prayer. Marc lets her put her palm against his chest, just left of centre where the heart is, then covers her hand with his own and presses it gently against him. Yes, he is saying. You can. Feel the heart. Sue closes her eyes and breathes deeply.

'Yeah, it's a very special thing, for Marc to feel it's okay for me to do this.'

They are both still for a moment, as she keeps her eyes closed and concentrates, then a smile spreads across Sue's face. She's beaming. Under her flat palm she can feel the warmth of his body and under that, the heart of her lost boy. The rhythm of life, the double thump as if it is repeating the name of her son, over and over again: Martin. Martin. Martin. The heart that grew in her womb. The heart Martin was born with and that kept him alive for sixteen years, always beating, unseen, on all the days she could remember. The day he took his first steps. The day he wouldn't let go of her hand at the school gate. The day he fell down in the park and she picked him up and hugged the hurt away. The heart was always there, always constant. Always beating. At home on the sofa, on that last night together, as they chatted and laughed, the heart was in him and he was alive.

Then he was gone.

The ache is still so hard to bear, it catches her breath after all this time, but now, here, under her fingertips, she can feel the rhythm that was his. A beat that began within her and grew louder in him and is now, some-how, still carrying on, impossibly, under the thin, scarred skin of this other boy. This man. 'That is really special to me,' says Sue slowly, her hand still in place like a blessing. 'To be able to feel the heart that Martin was born with, still beating … it's just incredible.'

This is not a quick grab of the hand. It's a moment that lingers, with a silence that grows. They are hip-to-hip on the sofa, the Scottish lad startled by the emotion of it all and the Englishwoman leaning across him, almost in an embrace. Almost like mother and son. Almost, but not quite. This is a rare kind of closeness that so few people can ever know, because the circumstances are so extraordinary. She lost her son and then his body was divided up. She survived a powerful grief and learned at last to let him go but now, incredibly, all these years later, she can feel for herself that a part of him is so very much alive. And Marc can feel this stranger close. He can feel her hand on him and his heart beating under it and yet he knows that the heart was not always his. It belonged to a boy who was – and is – so deeply loved by his mum, this woman whose hair is in Marc's face, whose scent is in his nostrils. No wonder they are both quiet. What could anyone say to all of that? A nervous little chuckle comes out of nowhere, surprising Marc. Sue echoes him and they shuffle apart, each looking happy but far away, shocked by what has just happened.

'I don't think you are actually aware of your own heart,' says Sue for something to say, nerves quickening her speech. 'You might hear it sometimes but not often and we rarely touch other people like this. I could feel Marc's heart beating strongly. For that, I'm really grateful.'

It's only when she gets up to make another mug of tea for us all that I realise I've just heard Sue call it Marc's heart. The heart that used to belong to the boy she misses every day. The loud, cheeky, lovely boy she lost far too soon, but whose death brought life. Martin, the boy who gave his heart away.

MARC & MARTIN

'This is not the way the world is meant to work. They're not supposed to go before us.'

That is what Linda said when she first thought her son was dying, all those years ago. She says it again now, when she calls to tell me that Marc has passed away.

'He died in my arms, Cole. I held him and he left me.'

Then the only sound down the line is sobbing.

This is not the way it is meant to be. The last time I saw Marc he was with Sue and looked so happy, so full of the promise of life to come. But that was in December 2015 and Linda says he went downhill fast in the following months. His heart began to struggle after thirteen years in a different body. His liver and kidneys began to fail again. He had a problem with his lungs and was diagnosed with a perforated bowel as well, so his visits to hospital became more frequent. Not that he would admit that he was dying, says his father.

'Marc came down to my house rubbing his side. I asked him what was wrong, and he said, "Oh Dad, I drunk too much milk today." It was nothing to do with milk. Even when I went to see him in hospital he'd be saying, "Dad, they don't know what they're talking about. What am I in for anyway?" What a boy. Unbelievable. I never left feeling sad. He lifted you up and kept you going, even though he knew how serious it all was.'

We did make a radio documentary about the transplant and it was broadcast that summer. Listeners rejoiced at Marc's recovery, but those who saw him every day knew he was in trouble. Despite being only twenty-eight years old, he moved about like a frail elderly man, unable to walk far. In July, at the height of summer with everybody enjoying the sun, Marc sat in yet another hospital room with his mother and a consultant told them both the bad news. There was nothing much more they could do for him. 'If they gave him a kidney transplant, his heart wouldn't cope. If they gave him a heart transplant, his kidneys wouldn't cope. The anaesthetic would kill him either way. We were between the devil and the deep blue sea,' says Linda. 'The doctor said he had two years to live, at the most. In the end we had two months.'

They wanted to go away together as a family one last time, so the heart and lung charity at the Freeman Hospital helped Linda arrange a weekend in September at a holiday camp in Whitley Bay, Northumberland, with an indoor pool and wide, sandy beaches. Marc insisted on driving his mum and a couple of his friends all the way. 'He was exhausted when we got there, but he was proud to have made it.'

More than a dozen of his friends and family were with him in a couple of caravans. They all feared it was his last holiday. A photograph taken that weekend shows Marc raising a vivid blue Slush Puppy ice drink alongside his brother's beer. He looks horribly pale and alarmingly thin. When they all left on the Monday morning, Marc was suffering severe stomach cramps again but still wanted to drive. They got as far as the border with Scotland before Linda had to take over.

'Shall I drive you straight to the hospital?'

'What for? 'Cos I'm tired? Ach no, Mum. I'll be fine.'

'You're not fine, son,' she said. But he insisted on going home to the house he was now sharing with his brother Darren. Marc texted his mum at 10.40 pm to say he felt better now he was in his own bed. But he also texted his sister, Leasa, and was straight with her.

'I'm away to the hospital in the morning. I'm fucked.'

'There's no harm in getting a wee help to make you better,' she texted back.

'I think I need a big help.'

When Leasa sent another message at seven the next morning to see how he was it was Darren who replied. He had found Marc unconscious on the bathroom floor just after five and called an ambulance. Leasa knew then that it was all over. 'If it had to happen, I'm glad it was only two months after he was told. I wouldn't have wanted him sitting there not able to move, counting down the days, not knowing what to say.'

Marc was taken to a state-of-the art hospital in Glasgow called the Queen Elizabeth, which had a new kind of scanner. Linda got there just after nine in the morning and found Marc in a cubicle in A&E with the curtains pulled all the way round it. She heard him first, because he was calling out for her and thrashing about like he had in the back of the car outside the hospital, long ago.

'Mum! I'm sore, Mum …'

'It's all right, baby, I'm here,' she said, but Linda saw the agony on his face and the heart monitor going crazy and she knew this really was the end of his life for sure, and she shrieked at the nurse. 'He's in pain here, give him something!'

The drugs calmed him down, as she recalls. 'Marc just pure relaxed and I just cuddled into him. His face was in my hair.'

After a while, a female doctor about the same age as Linda asked her to step outside the cubicle so they could talk. 'Your son is really very poorly,' she said.

'I know that, I've had thirteen years of it.'

Marc had suffered a heart attack and there was a build-up of fluid in his bowel, his life was under threat. They could operate but Linda knew it would probably kill him. They could resuscitate him if his heart failed again, but his mum did not want them to do that either. 'I didn't want my child dying on an operating table surrounded by strange people. And if they did resuscitate him, what would they be bringing him back for? To say, "Marc, you've got a perforated bowel but there's nothing we can do for you"? That would be cruel. So I said, "No, don't do those things. You are not to touch him anymore. Let him be."'

'You had better come back in,' said a nurse, interrupting. Marc was in trouble, he was having another heart attack. Linda threw her arms out as if to clear the space and ordered them not to intervene. 'Get all this stuff off him, all these sticky pads, the wires, the mask, the drips, everything. Leave me alone with my boy!'

The nurse and the doctor were brilliant, they did just that. Linda remembered what Leasa had told her a dozen years ago in Newcastle, that she should not cry when he was in trouble or it would frighten him. She was determined that Marc would not know that he was about to die. She got half up on the bed and cuddled him, cradling her son, stroking his hair, wetting his lips with her finger, rocking him.

'It's okay, son. It's okay. I'm here with you. I love you, baby, it's okay.'

She could hear the air coming out of his lungs. It was a sound she knew as a nurse, from the patients she had seen pass away. Then Linda says she felt a hand rubbing her back. The doctor was by her side, trying to comfort her. The nurse was on the other side. They both had their arms around her. The doctor placed a stethoscope on Marc's chest and listened.

'Linda, he's gone.'

Marc died in his mother's arms at 10.25 am on Tuesday, 20 September 2016. Linda stayed with him for the next five hours, in a private side room, while his family and friends came to say goodbye.

'It's strange, I could feel him watching us from somewhere – above, behind, I don't know – even while his body was lying there.'

She called an undertaker to fetch him, rather than have Marc go to the hospital mortuary, and even then she was talking to him. 'Look, son, I'm fighting for you.'

Daryl arrived at the hospital thinking Marc was still alive, but found his sister Leasa mumbling through tears. 'At least he's not suffering any more.'

'What do you mean?'

'Do you not know? He's away ...'

Daryl posted a message for all their friends and family on his Facebook timeline at 2.38 pm that afternoon: 'Just to let everyone know, my brother Marc passed away today. After a long 13-year fight dealing with a heart transplant, today his body finally had enough. He was a great uncle, brother, son, nephew, grandson and best mate to anyone who knew him. He will be missed dearly.'

Linda went to see his body at the funeral parlour on the Friday and said afterwards that she had been reminded of something Sue had said. 'I keep thinking about Marc being with Martin now. Like Martin has been waiting for him for thirteen years. Now they'll finally get to meet. He'll have a friend up there.'

* * *

Rangers flags and scarves have appeared overnight on walls and fences or hanging from the street lights all over Lochwinnoch, put there by friends of Marc wanting to 'turn the town blue' in his honour. The cloud is low, it's a grey and threatening day, with lashes of rain and the car headlights burning bright in the gloom. Nigel and Sue Burton have arrived an hour before the funeral service and are taking shelter in the Junction cafe, eating thick soup and crusty bread after their long journey. The drive up to Scotland took Nigel six hours and he will be driving six hours back, but they both felt compelled to come.

'We wanted to be with the family, but also we felt we needed to be here because they are burying a piece of Martin,' says Sue, dressed in a black coat and a black, white and blue dress. The men have been asked to wear a dark suit and a blue tie and Nigel's marks him out as a member of the Grantham Referees' Association, although nobody in Lochwinnoch is going to know that. They are with Lynne Holt, who has travelled by train all the way from Newcastle. Outside, the street is busy with people moving slowly towards the dark, solemn building that is Calder United Free Church.

The Burtons are quiet as they enter. The pews are already packed with Marc's friends and family, including lots of straight-backed lads with razored hair. The young women are elegant in black. They all look shocked into silence.

The front two rows of the church are empty, waiting for the close family.

We find seats to the side, and contemplate this place. The church was built by a congregation that believed in modesty in all things but the village was famous at the time for its furniture, and so the pulpit and the stairs leading up to it are beautifully made, somehow both simple and magnificent. The walls are white, the wood has been painted a warm gold. The sound of a piper playing in the street outside spills into the church. Heads turn to see Marc's coffin wheeled in through the door on a silver-looking trolley, to a stunned silence. The coffin is in the blue and white of the Scottish Saltire and bears a bouquet in the Rangers colours of red, white and blue. Marc is to be buried in a full Rangers kit – the socks, the shorts and the shirt all brand new. But the McCays are still not with us as the minister clicks his laptop to play the opening piano chords of a song called 'Faded' by Alan Walker.

'You were the shadow to my light. Did you feel us? Another star, you fade away. Where are you now?'

A lone, clear female voice sings but then a mighty wave of electronic dance music crashes in to the church, incongruous. Marc's mates would jump to their feet and start dancing if they heard that sound in a club, but instead they sit motionless in the pews, looking down at the floor.

Still, the family does not arrive.

The song cuts off abruptly and the minister comes to the microphone. 'Don't worry, folks, but are Nigel and Sue with us?' They are both confused to be picked out – but they get up and go out into a back room of the church as he directs. Linda is waiting. She wants Sue with her, for perhaps the most difficult moment of her life.

'We're burying Martin's heart. I can't do it without you.'

When the mothers have hugged, the close family group goes out into the church to take their places. Linda sits in the front pew, grasping hard at the hand of a longtime friend called Danny, a patient, supportive man who has become her partner in recent years. She slumps forward, face hidden behind her hair.

The minister carries on talking over her head, telling stories about Marc growing up in this community, going to Sunday school in this church, swimming in the river across the way, playing by the waterfall in the woods. 'He was a lively boy who once tied his little brother up and locked him in a cupboard.' Everyone laughs except Daryl – the little brother, now grown into a handsome young man – who has his own sad, secret smile.

Sparky – as they all seem to know Marc – took up a job cutting grass but the boss thought he spent more time kipping in the back of the van than working. He did get to play football with his brothers. They went with him to see Rangers play at Ibrox and the minister recalls that he even had calls from his great hero, the striker and manager Ally McCoist, who had heard his story. Then he asks us to sing the hymn so often heard at cup finals, 'Abide with Me'. The words are lovely, inspirational and reassuring, but the singing is thin. Throats are choked by emotion.

The minister mentions Martin and the heart that saved Marc's life, giving him thirteen more years, and says the McCays are profoundly grateful to the Burtons. 'The family would like to express their heartfelt thanks for that loving gift.' He reads a passage of promises from the Book of Jeremiah in the Bible, which ends with the words: 'I have loved you with a love that is everlasting.'

Now Daryl steps up to the microphone, swallows hard, blows out his cheeks and begins to read a poem by a friend about Marc:

> 'He was chosen to carry another boy's beat.
> He lived like a winner, never accepting defeat ...'

And it is time for the coffin to leave, to the sound of a song called 'See You Again' by Wiz Khalifa, which begins with piano and another sweet, lone voice. *'It's been a long day without you my friend and I'll tell you all about it when I see you again.'* And in the pause at the end of the line, Linda cries out in grief and pitches forward once more. She is held up by Danny, as the coffin begins to move.

The grave is open like a wound on the slope of the hill at Lochwinnoch Cemetery, a quiet and beautiful place on the edge of the village. The wind whispers in the high surrounding trees as hundreds of mourners gather in the rain. When everyone is in place, the funeral directors take their places with the coffin and hand silvered ropes to Leasa and the brothers, so that they can help lower Marc into the ground. The boys and his lifelong best friend, John, take turns to throw blue roses down after him. Each stands there in turn at the foot of the grave, not quite knowing what to do in the moment when a soldier would salute his fallen comrade.

Then Norrie, looking bewildered. He lets his flower drop.

Linda has a red rose she is holding to her face, breathing in the scent, cradling it like a baby. When her moment comes, she just can't let it go. The minister begins to say the words of the committal: 'Earth to earth, ashes to ashes, dust to dust …'

'No!'

Linda cries out. She stumbles into the arms of a friend. Then there is Sue, suddenly beside her, wrapping up Linda in her arms and holding her tight.

Now it is just the two of them, the mums alone together as if none of the rest of us are there at all. Sue's hand is on Linda's head, pressing it into her shoulder. They hold on to each other for a long time, by the graveside in the rain. The two mothers, unlikely friends, desperate allies. Each needs the other to help her stand.

Later, on the way out of the cemetery, Sue is asked if she is okay. 'No,' she says. 'Not really. It feels like burying Martin all over again.'

As evening comes, the mourners gather in the bar of the sports and social club in Lochwinnoch for sandwiches and sausage rolls, coffee or tea, pints or shots. Norrie takes me to one side and says that he listens to the radio series we made every night, when he gets in from work. 'I get myself a drink and I sit and listen, just to hear Marc's voice. I just want to hear the sound of my boy.'

The mothers sit together, eating very little, taking comfort in being with each other. 'I like your necklace,' says Sue, noticing Linda's silver pendant, a basket in the shape of a large heart with two hearts inside. Linda holds it up, for a better look. 'My friend gave it to me. She said the hearts belonged to Marc, Martin and me.'

Sue smiles and shows the two necklaces she also happens to be wearing, each in the shape of a heart. One is made from glittering diamanté. 'Marc gave me this, do you remember? In Canada, the first time we met?'

The other is a golden heart locket that she clicks open to show a picture of Martin. Thirteen years have passed since she bent to kiss him goodbye in the hospital for the last time, saying softly and fondly, 'Sleep tight. We'll love you forever.'

Now the heart that carried on beating for so long after his death has been put in the ground with Marc McCay and Sue feels the loss of her son all over again, as if it has only just happened. Linda shares her pain and searches for comfort, saying: 'They're up there together, helping each other out.' Maybe that's true. Maybe it's an echo of what is happening here, between the mothers. But even if they never see the boys again, both of these women have given their all to their sons and the words that were read out loud today will always be true.

'I have loved you with a love that is everlasting.'

FOR MARC
AND MARTIN

Thank you to Sue and Nigel Burton and Linda and Norrie McCay for telling their stories, and to Marc McCay for sharing so much. Thanks also to the wider McCay family, particularly Darren, Daryl, Ryan and Leasa. Harish Vyas, Leslie Hamilton and Lynne Holt were very generous with their time and patient in their attempts to explain. Any medical errors are mine, not theirs. I have tried to keep as closely as possible to what I was told by all concerned, with some changes for the sake of privacy or clarity. This account is not intended to imply mistakes or blame on the part of any individual or institution in any way. The NHS is a national treasure. Please consider registering as a donor and helping the charities overleaf:

www.donorfamilynetwork.co.uk
www.organdonation.nhs.uk
www.transplantsport.org.uk

This edited quote from Henry Scott Holland, once Regius Professor of Divinity at Oxford University, was posted on Facebook by Linda McCay after Marc's death. The words were a comfort to her:

Whatever we were to each other, that we are still. Call me by the old familiar name. Speak of me in the easy way which you always used. Laugh as we always laughed at the little jokes that we enjoyed together. Play, smile, think of me, pray for me. Why should I be out of mind because I am out of sight? I am but waiting for you, for an interval, somewhere very near, just round the corner. All is well.

AUTHOR'S THANKS

Many thanks to Elizabeth Sheinkman at WME, Natalie Jerome and Zoe Berville at HarperCollins for their expert assistance in making this book happen. I'm also grateful to Jonathan Mayo, Rhian Roberts, Phil Critchlow, Mandy Appleyard and Rupert Lee for the various ways in which they helped me understand or shape the narrative. Thanks, always, to Rachel, Jacob, Joshua, Ruby and Grace.

Moving Memoirs

Stories of hope, courage and the power of love…

If you loved this book, then you will love our Moving Memoirs eNewsletter

Sign up to…

- Be the first to hear about new books

- Get sneak previews from your favourite authors

- Read exclusive interviews

- Be entered into our monthly prize draw to win one of our latest releases before it's even hit the shops!

Sign up at

www.moving-memoirs.com